Anatomy:
Review for USMLE, Step 1, Second Edition

Anatomy:
Review for USMLE, Step 1,
Second Edition

Kurt E. Johnson, Ph.D.
Professor of Anatomy and Cell Biology

Frank J. Slaby, Ph.D.
Associate Professor of Anatomy and Cell Biology

Ronald C. Bohn, Ph. D.
Associate Professor of Anatomy and Cell Biology

The George Washington University Medical Center
Washington, D.C.

J&S

J&S Publishing Company Inc., Alexandria, Virginia

J&S

Composition and Layout: Ronald C. Bohn, Ph.D.
Cover Design: Kurt E. Johnson, Ph.D.
Printing Supervisor: Robert Perotti, Jr.
Printing: Goodway Graphics of Virginia, Inc., Springfield, VA

Library of Congress Catalog Card Number 98-065379

ISBN 1-888308-03-6

Dedication

Kurt E. Johnson would like to dedicate his portion of this book to his wife, Julie M. Okkema, M.D. and his children, Melissa, Abraham, Justine, and Alexander. Frank J. Slaby would like to dedicate his portion of this book to his wife Susan K. McCune, M.D. and their son Christopher. Ronald C. Bohn would like to dedicate his portion of this book to his wife Susan and their son Eric.

Table of Contents

Preface to First Edition

This book is designed to enable you to review in just 1-2 days all of the basic anatomical sciences you studied in the first year of medical school: Cell Biology and Histology, Embryology, Gross Anatomy and Neuroanatomy. We have been able to condense a review of all basic anatomical sciences into a single book because of the new format of the National Board Part I Exam. It is no longer prudent to review exhaustively the basic science courses because the new examination format no longer rewards an encyclopedic knowledge of the basic sciences. Instead, the new exams test knowledge of the scientific basis of disease and injury and the ability to apply basic scientific information to the clinical reasoning process. Consequently, the most efficient way to study for the new exam is 1) to review only the most clinically relevant material from each basic science course and 2) to focus on the application of this material to the solution of clinical problems. These two new study features form the core of this text.

If you answer every question and read all the tutorials in this book, you can cover within 2 days all of the most clinically relevant information from your basic anatomical science courses. You will find that many anatomical facts reviewed or learned anew will be presented in the context of a clinical case or an illustration. We hope that the clinical cases and illustrations will enhance your understanding and recall of the information. Finally, you will learn from the tutorials how anatomical information is used by knowledgeable physicians to understand the courses of diseases, the mechanisms of injuries and the significance of abnormal findings.

Kurt E. Johnson, Ph.D.
Frank J. Slaby, Ph.D.
Washington, D.C.
April, 1992

Preface to Second Edition

We approached production of **Anatomy: Review for USMLE, Step 1, Second Edition** *with trepidation. We were stunned and gratified by the acceptance of the first edition of our little book. The second edition retains the substance and spirit of the first edition but departs from it in the following ways:*

1)   We have replaced some simple matching items with extended matching items.
2)   Some of the tutorials have been fleshed out a bit
3)   We have replaced some simple items with clinical scenarios followed by items to reflect the growing clinical emphasis of the USMLE, Step 1.
4)   We have replaced some of the supernumerary karyotypes with patient photographs and clinically-oriented items.

We sincerely hope that you will find that this new iteration as useful as your predecessors found the first edition. Good luck on your examinations.

Kurt E. Johnson, Ph. D.
Frank J. Slaby, Ph. D.
Ronald C. Bohn, Ph. D.
Washington, D.C.
February, 1998

Acknowledgements

The authors would like to thank Ronald C. Bohn, Ph.D., Associate Professor, Department of Anatomy and Cell Biology, The George Washington University Medical Center for his skillful work in formatting the final documents for publication. We would also like to thank Mark R. Adelman, Ph.D., Associate Professor, Department of Anatomy, Uniformed Services University of the Health Sciences for reading and correcting Chapters I and II. We would like to acknowledge the use of the excellent illustrations by Diane Abeloff, A.M.I. published in **Medical Art: Graphics for Use**, *Williams and Wilkins, Baltimore, 1982. We would also like to thank Raymond J. Walsh, Ph.D., Professor and Chairman, Department of Anatomy, George Washington University Medical Center for his support of this project.*

Disclaimer

The clinical information presented in this book is accurate for the purposes of review for licensure examinations but in no way should be used to treat patients or substituted for modern clinical training. Proper diagnosis and treatment of patients requires comprehensive evaluation of all symptoms, careful monitoring for adverse responses to treatment and assessment of the long-term consequences of therapeutic intervention.

CHAPTER I
HISTOLOGY AND CELL BIOLOGY

Items 1-5

For each statement of structure, function or embryological origin in the items below, select the **MOST** appropriate structure in **Figure 1.1**. Answers may be used once, more than once, or not at all.

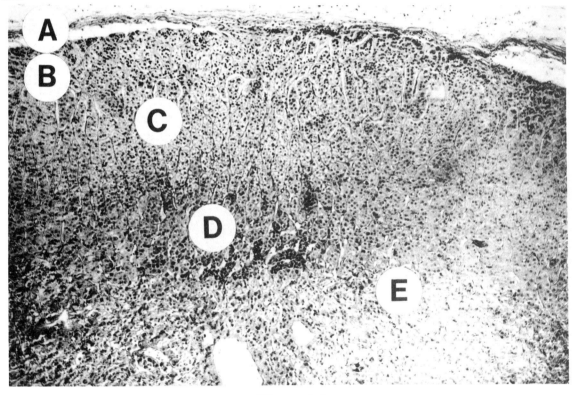

Figure 1.1

1. This structure is derived from the neural crest.

2. This structure has cells with abundant smooth endoplasmic reticulum, mitochondria with tubular cristae, and especially large lipid droplets.

3. This structure secretes mineralocorticoids.

4. This structure secretes sex steroids and is derived from the lining of the primitive coelomic cavity.

5.   Epithelial cells in this structure are arranged in long straight cords running parallel to long straight sinusoids.

ANSWERS AND TUTORIAL ON ITEMS 1-5

The answers are: **1-E; 2-C; 3-B; 4-D; 5-C**. **Figure 1.1** is a photomicrograph of the human adrenal gland. It is surrounded by a thin **connective tissue capsule** (A). The **adrenal cortex** (B-D) arises from proliferation of the mesodermally derived coelomic epithelium and consists of three layers of cells. The outer layer is the **zona glomerulosa** (B). It is a source of mineralocorticoids. The middle and thickest layer is the **zona fasciculata** (C). It consists of long, straight cords of epithelial cells arranged between long sinusoids. The cortical cells all have an abundance of smooth endoplasmic reticulum and mitochondria with tubular cristae, ultrastructural features common to all steroid secreting cells. The cells of the zona fasciculata have a foamy appearance in the light microscope due to a profusion of large lipid rich vacuoles. The cells of the zona fasciculata secrete glucocorticoids. The cells of the **zona reticularis** (D) secrete sex steroids. The **adrenal medulla** (E) is derived from the neural crest and consists of two populations of secretory cells, one secreting epinephrine and the other secreting norepinephrine.

Match the cell type in the answers below with its **MOST** appropriate description in the items below. Answers may be used once, more than once, or not at all.

> (A)   Lactotropes
> (B)   Gonadotropes
> (C)   Corticotropes
> (D)   Thyrotropes
> (E)   Somatotropes

6.   These acidophils are found in the pars distalis. When they are hyperactive in adults, acromegaly results.

7.   These basophils secrete luteinizing hormone and follicle-stimulating hormone.

8.   Adrenalectomy would result in degranulation of these cells due to release of ACTH.

ANSWERS AND TUTORIAL ON ITEMS 6-8

The answers are: **6-E; 7-B; 8-C**. All of these cell types are found in the **adenohypophysis** of the **pituitary gland**. **Corticotropes** (large granules), **gonadotropes** (medium granules) and **thyrotropes** (small granules) are all basophils. **Lactotropes** and **somatotropes** are acidophils. Corticotropes secrete **ACTH** which in turn stimulates steroid secretion from the adrenal cortex. **Adrenalectomy** would remove the feedback inhibition of ACTH secretion and thus cause massive degranulation of corticotropes. Gonadotropes secrete FSH and LH (ICSH), hormones that are involved in the regulation of gamete formation in the gonads. Thyrotropes secrete **TSH** which stimulates thyroxine secretion in the thyroid gland. Lactotropes produce **prolactin** which stimulates development of the mammary glands and lactation. Somatotropes secrete **growth hormone**. Excessive secretion of growth hormone in adults leads to **acromegaly**.

Examine the high power light micrograph of a mature ovarian follicle in **Figure 1.2** below and then choose the **MOST** appropriate labeled structure to match the functional role or morphological description of this structure. Answers may be used once, more than once, or not at all.

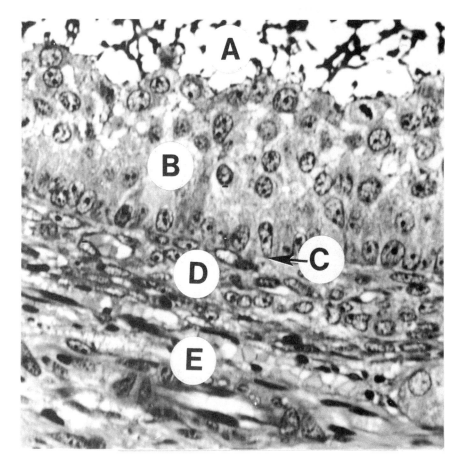

Figure 1.2

9.   This structure is rich in laminin and is the outer boundary of the follicular epithelium.

10.   These cells secrete androstenedione, an estradiol precursor.

11.   These cells secrete liquor folliculi and the zona pellucida before ovulation and steroids after ovulation.

ANSWERS AND TUTORIAL ON ITEMS 9-11

The answers are: **9-C; 10-D; 11-B**. **Figure 1.2** is a high magnification light micrograph of a portion of a mature ovarian follicle and the adjacent thecal and stromal cells associated with this follicle. The follicle is bounded by a **basement membrane** (C). Inside the basement membrane, there are several layers of **granulosa cells** (B). Not shown in this photograph is the oocyte surrounded by a group of granulosa cells known collectively as the **cumulus oophorus**. The granulosa cells are thought to be involved in supporting the development of the follicle in several ways. First, they proliferate and contribute to the growth of the follicle. Second, they secrete a viscous **liquor folliculi** (A) into a growing follicular antrum. Third, they secrete **estradiol** synthesized from androstenedione derived from the cells of the **theca interna** (D). The **theca externa** is also shown (E). After ovulation, the follicle is converted into a steroid secreting **corpus luteum**. The granulosa cells differentiate into **granulosa lutein cells** of the corpus luteum. The theca interna cells also contribute to the formation of the corpus luteum by differentiating into **theca lutein cells**. The steroids secreted by the developing follicle prior to ovulation stimulate the growth of endometrial glands. After ovulation, hormones of the corpus luteum stimulate the secretory activity of endometrial glands in preparation for implantation of the conceptus in the wall of the uterus.

Items 12-14

You encounter a patient who is phenotypically female. Karyotype analysis reveals a normal looking 46, XY karyotype. Molecular biological investigation of the Y chromosome DNA sequences shows a deletion of the SRY gene. Choose the **BEST** response.

12.   The SRY gene

      (A)   drives ovarian development
      (B)   encodes for an insulin-like growth factor
      (C)   is required for testicular development
      (D)   All of the above
      (E)   None of the above

13. If the patient had a 46, XX karyotype with the SRY region of the Y chromosome translocated into the X chromosome the patient would

    (A) be phenotypically female
    (B) be phenotypically male
    (C) be a hermaphrodite
    (D) have Turner's syndrome
    (E) have Klinefelter's syndrome

14. The SRY gene maps to

    (A) the short arm of the Y chromosome
    (B) the long arm of the Y chromosome
    (C) the short arm of the X chromosome
    (D) the long arm of the X chromosome
    (E) None of the above

ANSWERS AND TUTORIAL ON ITEMS 12-14

The answers are: **12-C; 13-B; 14-A**. The **SRY gene** product is a **transcription factor**. Some growth factors and oncogene products are also transcription factors. When the DNA sequence encoding the SRY is deleted from the Y chromosome, **sex reversal** results. A male karyotype and a female phenotype will occur. Conversely, when the DNA sequence encoding for the SRY is translocated from the Y chromosome to the X chromosome, sex reversal will result again. In this instance, a female karyotype and a male phenotype will be associated. The SRY is expressed specifically in the genital ridge mesenchyme immediately before the indifferent gonad becomes committed to testis formation. Thus, the SRY gene product drives the differentiation of the indifferent gonad in the male direction. Differentiation of a testis then directs further sexual differentiation in a male direction. **Turner's syndrome** is caused by a monosomy of the X chromosome (45, X). **Klinefelter's syndrome** is cause by aneuploidy of sex chromosomes (47, XXY).

Recent discoveries in developmental genetics reveal a connection between ß transforming growth factor (ß-TGF), nerve growth factor (NGF), homeodomain proteins, and the fos gene product. Choose the **BEST** response.

15.   All of these polypeptides

      (A)   are DNA polymerases
      (B)   are translation factors
      (C)   are transcription factors
      (D)   bind to mRNA
      (E)   block tRNA turnover

16.   Their chief mechanism of action is to

      (A)   promote specific mRNA synthesis
      (B)   inhibit DNA synthesis
      (C)   promote specific tRNA synthesis
      (D)   suppress gene expression
      (E)   activate genes for rRNA synthesis

17.   They are thought to result in differentiation by

      (A)   repression of gene expression
      (B)   controlling differential gene expression
      (C)   promoting turnover of the rough endoplasmic reticulum
      (D)   converting rough endoplasmic reticulum into smooth endoplasmic reticulum
      (E)   stimulation of mitochondrial DNA polymerase

ANSWERS AND TUTORIAL ON ITEMS 15-17

The answers are: **15-C; 16-A; 17-B**. ß-TGF, NGF, homeodomain proteins, and the fos gene product are all examples of **transcription factors**. They bind to DNA causing its uncoiling and promote its transcription into specific mRNAs. The action of these transcription factors is thought to represent the fundamental basis for **differential gene expression**. All cells in an organism are thought to have the same DNA complement. The formation of the multiple differentiated cell types within an organism, e.g., neurons, muscle cells and liver cells, is due to selective activation of some subset of genes within the precursor of that individual cell type. Once these genes are activated by transcription factors, specific transcription and translation results in the formation of an array of proteins peculiar to that highly differentiated cell type.

Experimental vascular perfusion of the testis with lanthanum nitrate (an electron dense, low molecular weight tracer) is followed by fixation of seminiferous tubules. Subsequently, seminiferous tubules are prepared for transmission electron microscopy. Choose the **BEST** response.

18. Lanthanum nitrate would be found in all of the following anatomical locations **EXCEPT**:

    (A) interstitial tissue
    (B) surrounding Leydig cells
    (C) around primordial germ cells
    (D) around immature primary spermatocytes
    (E) around spermatids

19. What anatomical structural arrangement prevents penetration of lanthanum nitrate into the adluminal compartment?

    (A) desmosomes
    (B) zonula adherens
    (C) tight junctions
    (D) gap junctions
    (E) the basement membrane of the seminiferous epithelium

20. These structural elements also function in the formation of all of the following morphological barriers **EXCEPT**:

    (A) blood-urine barrier in kidney
    (B) blood-brain barrier
    (C) blood-bile barrier
    (D) impermeable continuous capillaries
    (E) barrier preventing leakage of digestive enzymes from intestinal lumen

ANSWERS AND TUTORIAL ON ITEMS 18-20

The answers are: **18-E; 19-C; 20-A. Tight junctions** are an essential feature of many epithelial layers. Epithelia line cavities and cover surfaces. They have tight lateral junctions that allow them to serve as boundary tissues, separating one compartment in the body from another. For example, intestinal epithelial cells are joined together by apical junctional complexes. The **junctional complex** consists of an apical **zonula occludens** or tight junction, a **zonula adherens** just deep to the zonula occludens and a **macula adherens** (desmosome) deep to the zonula adherens. The tight junction is a region of fusion of the outer leaflets of the plasma membranes of adjacent cells. It provides a hydrophobic barrier preventing the contents of the intestinal lumen (digestive enzymes) from diffusing into the lateral spaces between cells. Tight junctions are also present between capillary endothelial cells in continuous capillaries where they serve as the anatomical basis for the blood-brain barrier and between liver parenchymal cells where they serve as the anatomical basis for the blood-bile barrier.

The blood-urine barrier in the kidney is more complex. The glomerular basement membrane and the filtration slit diaphragms between podocyte foot processes serve as the anatomical barrier between blood and urine.

In the seminiferous epithelium, **Sertoli cells** form a continuous epithelial layer. The spermatogenic cell line is lodged in the spaces between Sertoli cells. A complex web of tight junctions between adjacent Sertoli cells divides the seminiferous epithelium into a **basal compartment** containing only spermatogonia, preleptotene primary spermatocytes and leptotene primary spermatocytes. Later stages in spermatogenesis including late primary spermatocytes, secondary spermatocytes, spermatids and spermatozoa are contained within the **adluminal compartment** apical to the web of tight junctions. This elaborate system of tight junctions prevents exposure of foreign antigens of mature gametes to the immune system. During fetal development, the male gonad becomes equipped with spermatogonia prior to the time in development when the immune system gains the ability to discriminate between native and foreign antigens. Thus, spermatogonia are recognized as native antigens. Spermatogenesis does not begin until puberty, long after the establishment of the immunological sense of native and foreign antigens. Consequently, the surface antigens peculiar to spermatozoa would be recognized as foreign antigens were it not for the tight junctions excluding these foreign antigens from immune surveillance. Robust junctional complexes between epithelial cells lining the excurrent testicular ducts (e.g., efferent ductules, epididymis, ductus deferens, and prostate gland) also limit contact between seminal antigens and the male circulatory system.

9

Items 21-24

Examine the labeled photomicrograph of a developing bone of the appendicular skeleton in **Figure 1.3** below. Match the lettered structure in the photomicrograph with the **MOST** appropriate description of its developmental fate or role in endochondral bone formation in the items. Answers may be used once, more than once, or not at all.

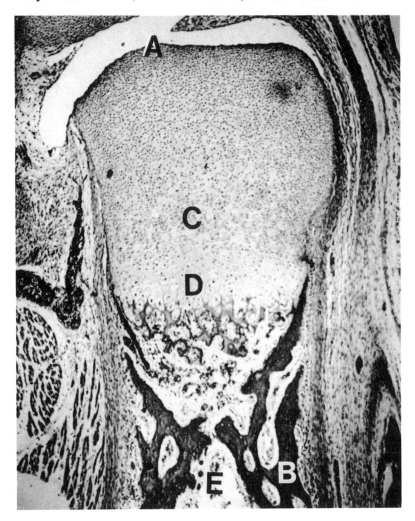

Figure 1.3

21.   This structure represents an active site of osteoid deposition.

22.   This region contains many mitotically active chondrocytes.

23.   This region contains hypertrophic chondrocytes.

24.   This region persists as hyaline cartilage even adult bones.

ANSWERS AND TUTORIAL ON ITEMS 21-24

The answers are: **21-B; 22-C; 23-D; 24-A**. All bones of the appendicular skeleton as well as vertebrae, the base of the skull, ribs and the sternum are formed by the ossification of cartilaginous models of these bones. This type of bone formation is called **endochondral bone formation**. The bones of the vault of the skull and certain facial bones are formed spontaneously in mesenchyme without a pre-existing cartilaginous model by **intramembranous bone formation** (**Figure 1.3**). During endochondral bone formation, the cartilaginous model grows by mitotic proliferation of chondrocytes in the **zone of proliferation** (C) or by addition of new chondrocytes to the outer surface of the growing cartilaginous model. Certain mesenchymal cells in the future metaphysis of the bone differentiate into osteoblasts. These cells secrete an extracellular matrix characteristic of bone which calcifies rapidly, forming a **bony collar** (B) around the cartilage. The nutrient supply of chondrocytes is restricted by the bony collar and they therefore undergo **hypertrophy** (D) and then degenerate and die, leading to the formation of a **marrow cavity** (E). Meanwhile, growth continues in the zone of proliferation. New cartilage is rapidly converted into bone. Once the final size of the bone has been established at puberty, further proliferation of the cartilage is not possible. The hyaline cartilage on the **articular surface** (A) of these bony models persists as the articular cartilage.

Items 25-27

For each component of the junctional complex below, select the **MOST** appropriate associated functional role of this component. Answers may be used once, more than once, or not at all.

> (A) Zonula occludens
> (B) Zonular adherens
> (C) Macula adherens
> (D) Gap junction
> (E) Microfilaments

25. This is a location where aqueous channels between cells assure free intercellular passage of small molecules.

26. This structure is thought to be involved in intercellular adhesions. Here one finds dense plaques on the cytoplasmic face of apposed membranes which serve as insertion sites for tonofilaments.

27. This is a site of fusion of outer leaflets of the plasma membrane. It is a tight junction preventing luminal materials from leaving the lumen.

ANSWERS AND TUTORIAL ON ITEMS 25-27

The answers are: **25-D; 26-C; 27-A**. **Epithelial tissue** defines boundaries and establishes compartments in the human body. For example, the lumen of the small intestine contains a complicated mixture of digestive enzymes capable of digesting the wall of the small intestine. The contents of the lumen of the GI tract are isolated from the sensitive wall of the gut by a membrane specialization known as the **junctional complex**. At the most apical portion of the junctional complex there is a **tight junction** where the outer leaflets of the membranes fuse into an occluding junction called the **zonula occludens**. This structure extends belt-like around the apex of the columnar epithelial cells and makes a seal between the lumen and the lateral extracellular fluid environment. In freeze-fracture-etch, the zonula occludens sometimes occurs as an anastomosing network of ridges (points of membrane fusion) representing multiple barriers to movement of molecules from the lumen to the lateral extracellular compartment. Below the zonula occludens there is a divergence of the plasma membrane with a clear separation of 10 to 15 nm. This structure is called the **zonula adherens**. There is simple membrane apposition with variable amounts of electron dense material in the intervening 10-15 nm gap. Numerous 6 nm **microfilaments** radiate away from the zonula adherens into the cytoplasmic matrix of apposed cells. This structure is usually described as an adhesive junction. The **macula adherens** (desmosome) is found below the zonula adherens. At the macula adherens, the plasma membranes diverge to 25-30 nm. There is an intermediate dense line running between the cells. On the inner face of each apposed plasma membrane there is a plaque of electron dense material. Long bundles of 10 nm intermediate filaments called **tonofilaments** radiate away from the plaque of electron dense material. The macula adherens is thought to be a structure holding cells together. **Gap junctions** are also commonly associated with the junctional complex. In the gap junction (sometimes called a nexus), the outer leaflets of the membranes of adjacent cells approach to within 2 nm, but a small but definite gap remains. Gap junctions are composed of hexagonal arrays of barrel-shaped structures with six subunits arranged around a central core which is an aqueous channel between closely apposed cells, allowing the free passage of ions and other small molecules between epithelial cells.

12

Examine the transmission electron micrograph in **Figure 1.4** below and then choose the **BEST** answer. Answers may be used once, more than once, or not at all.

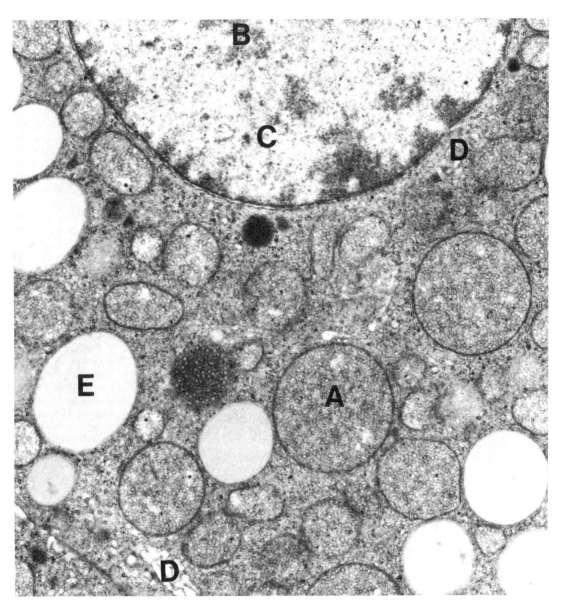

Figure 1.4

28. Which physiological function is most characteristic of a cell with this ultrastructure?

    (A)   mucus secretion
    (B)   zymogen granule production
    (C)   steroid synthesis
    (D)   glycogen storage
    (E)   motility

29. This kind of a cell would be most prominent in which anatomical location?

    (A)   gastric mucosa
    (B)   pancreatic acini
    (C)   adrenal cortex
    (D)   liver parenchyma
    (E)   wall of the urinary bladder

For each physiological function, select the **MOST** appropriate corresponding labeled structure in the transmission electron micrograph in **Figure 1.4**.

30. Site of storage of cholesterol esters, precursors for the steroid secretion products of this cell.

31. Produces ATP and is involved in steroid biosynthesis.

ANSWERS AND TUTORIAL ON ITEMS 28-31

The answers are: **28-C; 29-C; 30-E; 31-A**. **Figure 1.4** is a transmission electron micrograph of a cell from the **adrenal cortex**. It has an ultrastructure characteristic of cells secreting **steroids** including an abundance of **smooth endoplasmic reticulum** (D) (not well illustrated here), numerous **lipid droplets** (E), large round **mitochondria** (A) with tubulovesicular cristae and small dense bodies. The **nucleolus** (B) in the **nucleus** (C) is prominent. This cell synthesizes cortisol from cholesterol esters stored in **lipid droplets** (E). Cholesterol is released from the lipid droplets and enters mitochondria where it is converted into pregnenolone. In the smooth endoplasmic reticulum, pregnenolone is converted to progesterone and then 17-deoxycorticosterone, which is finally converted into cortisol by mitochondrial enzymes. The factors controlling the shuttling of different intermediates from lipid droplets to mitochondria to smooth endoplasmic reticulum and back to mitochondria are not well understood. Also, the mechanism of steroid secretion is controversial with most authors favoring direct release of steroids by diffusion. Steroid secreting cells are abundant in the adrenal cortex, in the corpus luteum, in the placenta and in the interstitium of the testis (Leydig cells).

Following a lipid rich meal, dietary lipids are processed and transported to the liver. Choose the **MOST** appropriate anatomical location for the physiological process described in the items below. Answers may be used once, more than once, or not at all.

          (A)   Lumen of intestine
          (B)   Microvilli
          (C)   Smooth endoplasmic reticulum of intestinal absorptive epithelial cell
          (D)   Golgi apparatus of intestinal absorptive epithelial cell
          (E)   Lacteals

32.   Chylomicra are synthesized from triglycerides, glycolipids and proteins.

33.   Free fatty acids and monoglycerides are converted into triglycerides.

34.   Chylomicra are transported via these lymphatic vessels to the systemic circulation.

ANSWERS AND TUTORIAL ON ITEMS 32-34

The answers are: **32-D; 33-C; 34-E**. Dietary fat, composed mainly of **triglycerides**, is hydrolyzed to fatty acids and monoglycerides in the lumen of the small intestine by the action of **lipases** secreted by the pancreas. Fatty acids and monoglycerides diffuse across the plasma membranes of intestinal microvilli and into the cisternae of the **smooth endoplasmic reticulum** located in the apical cytoplasm of absorptive cells. Here, the fatty acids and monoglycerides are resynthesized into triglycerides. Next, the triglycerides are transported to the **Golgi apparatus** where they are further processed by addition of glycolipids and proteins to form the **chylomicra**. Chylomicra are now expelled from the lateral borders of absorptive epithelial cells into intercellular spaces where they move across the epithelial basement membrane and finally enter the lumen of blind ending lymphatic capillaries (lacteals) in the core of intestinal villi. Lymphatic vessels conduct the chylomicra to the systemic circulation. The contraction of slips of smooth muscle in the villi probably aids in proximal transport of chylomicra.

Examine the labeled photomicrograph in **Figure 1.5** below and then match the lettered structure with the **MOST** appropriate description of its microscopic anatomy, developmental origins or physiological role. Answers may be used once, more than once, or not at all.

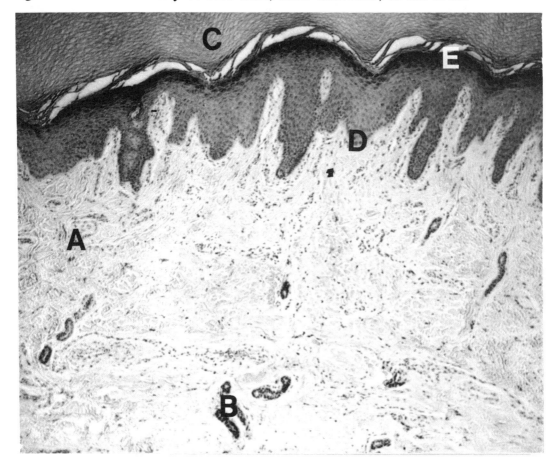

Figure 1.5

35. This structure is derived from segmentally-arranged dermomyotomes which are formed by proliferation in derivatives of the intraembryonic mesoderm.

36. This structure contains cells with nuclei protected on their apical side by a layer of melanin granules.

37. This structure contains undifferentiated stem cells that are mitotically active.

38. This structure functions to prevent desiccation of the body from within and contains cross-linked keratin forming a hydrophobic barrier.

39.   This structure is formed by invagination of ectodermal derivatives.

40.   This structure contains keratohyalin granules.

ANSWERS AND TUTORIAL ON ITEMS 35-40

The answers are: **35-A; 36-D; 37-D; 38-C; 39-B; 40-E. Figure 1.5** is a photomicrograph of human skin. It consists of an epithelial epidermis and a connective tissue **dermis** (A). The dermis is derived from a component of the somite known as the dermomyotome. **Somites** are segmentally-arranged structures forming in the intraembryonic mesoderm. The most basal layer of the epidermis is the **stratum germinativum** (D). It consists of undifferentiated stem cells capable of repeated rounds of mitosis to produce all of the more apical epidermal layers. Because these stems cells are mitotically active and exposed to mutagenic UV irradiation from the sun, their nuclei are capped with melanin granules that absorb UV rays. The **stratum granulosum** (E) is intermediate between the deep stratum germinativum and the superficial **stratum corneum** (C). The stratum granulosum contains basophilic keratohyalin granules that contribute components to the keratinization process. The stratum corneum consists of many layers of dry, dead squamous cells. Each cell contains a high concentration of keratin, a highly cross-linked protein made up of many hydrophobic amino acids. This layer prevents unwanted substances from entering the body and also prevents loss of interstitial water. An **eccrine sweat gland** (B) is also shown. It is formed by invagination of the surface ectoderm deep into the dermis. Surface ectoderm eventually differentiates into the epidermis and all epidermal appendages including sweat glands, sebaceous glands, hair, eyelashes and nails under the inductive influence of underlying dermal connective tissues.

Examine the scanning electron micrographs in **Figure 1.6** below. The area in the box in the left micrograph is shown at higher magnification in the right micrograph. Match the structure in the micrograph with the **MOST** appropriate description of its microscopic anatomy or physiological role. Answers may be used once, more than once, or not at all.

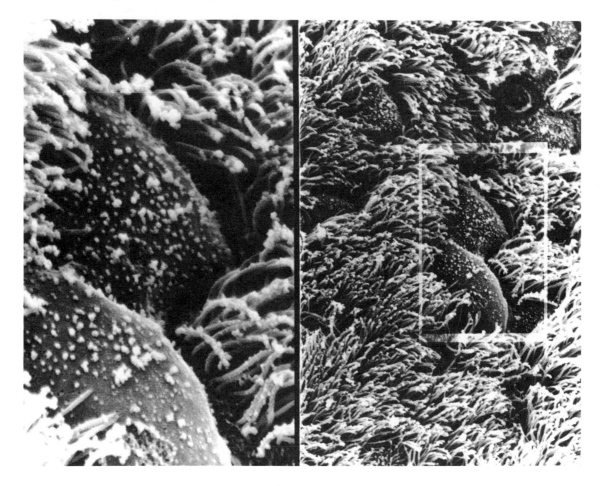

Figure 1.6

41.   The **BEST** functional description of the two cells inside the box is

(A)   Their secretion product has a digestive function.
(B)   Their secretion product traps inspired debris.
(C)   Their secretion product moistens ingested food.
(D)   They are involved in absorption of materials from the lumen of this organ.
(E)   They are involved in excretion of urea.

42. The **BEST** microanatomical description of the predominant cell type in this micrograph is

    (A) abundant smooth endoplasmic reticulum and mitochondria with tubular cristae
    (B) abundant rough endoplasmic reticulum and many zymogen granules
    (C) basal bodies and apical mitochondria
    (D) basal infoldings and basal mitochondria
    (E) apical microvilli

43. The **MOST** abundant and physiologically significant cytoskeletal element in the predominant cell type is

    (A) actin-containing microfilaments
    (B) desmin-containing intermediate filaments
    (C) keratin-containing intermediate filaments
    (D) vimentin-containing intermediate filaments
    (E) dynein-containing microtubular pairs

44. Both kinds of cells would be found in all of the following anatomical locations **EXCEPT**:

    (A) uterus
    (B) uterine tubes
    (C) trachea
    (D) bronchi
    (E) terminal bronchioles

ANSWERS AND TUTORIAL ON ITEMS 41-44

The answers are: **41-B; 42-C; 43-E; 44-E. Figure 1.6** is a scanning electron micrograph of the apical surface of the human **tracheal epithelium**. The apical layer of this pseudostratified epithelium consists mainly of abundant **ciliated cells** (the predominant cell type in the photomicrograph) and sparse **goblet cells** (in the box). Goblet cells secrete a thick mucus that traps inspired debris in the respiratory system. Ciliated cells have many **cilia** consisting of nine peripheral doublets of **microtubules** and a central pair of microtubules. **Dynein** is an ATPase attached to the microtubules and is required for ciliary movement. The apical cytoplasm of ciliated cells contains basal bodies (modified centrioles) for anchoring cilia and an abundance of mitochondria for producing ATP to drive ciliary beating. Basal cells (stem cells) and brush cells are also found in the tracheal epithelium.

      Mixtures of ciliated cells and goblet cells are found in much of the female reproductive tract including the uterine tubes and uterus and in the portions of the respiratory system proximal to the terminal bronchioles such as the trachea, bronchi and bronchioles. Terminal bronchioles have ciliated cells but lack goblet cells.

Examine the transmission electron micrograph in **Figure 1.7** below. Match the labeled structure in the micrograph with the **MOST** appropriate description of its microscopic anatomy or physiological role. Answers may be used once, more than once, or not at all.

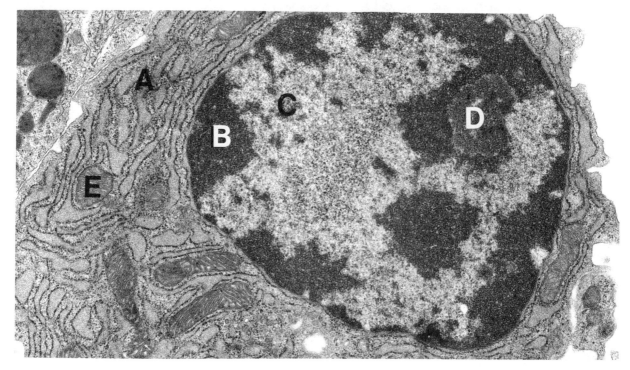

Figure 1.7

45. These contain nascent polypeptide chains destined for exocytosis.

46. These contain enzymes for the electron transport chain of oxidative phosphorylation.

47. This structure contains the DNA which encodes ribosomal RNA.

48. This cell is a

    (A) neutrophil
    (B) macrophage
    (C) plasma cell
    (D) lymphocyte
    (E) mast cell

49. The chief secretion product of this cell is

    (A) lipase
    (B) α-amylase
    (C) immunoglobulin
    (D) transferrin
    (E) lactoperoxidase

Items 50-52

A 55-year-old alcoholic male shows hemorrhages near the base of hair follicles and swollen gingivae around his teeth. He has cutaneous lesions that have healed poorly. A fractured toe has not healed properly after 3 months. Histological examination of the lesions reveals extensive granulation tissue with few collagen fibers. A diagnosis of scurvy is made. Choose the **BEST** response.

50. The cells **MOST** affected in scurvy are

    (A) liver parenchymal cells
    (B) osteoclasts
    (C) fibroblasts
    (D) plasma cells
    (E) eosinophils

51. Scurvy is the result of a defect in

    (A) elastin biosynthesis
    (B) tropocollagen biosynthesis
    (C) collagen cross-linking
    (D) laminin polymerization
    (E) fibronectin binding

52. The **MOST** accurate description of the fundamental lesion involved in the etiology of this dietary deficiency is

    (A) deficient synthesis of collagen alpha chains
    (B) leakage of capillaries
    (C) decreased cross-linkage at desmosyl residues
    (D) increased hydrolysis of tropocollagen telopeptides
    (E) increased collagen turnover

ANSWERS AND TUTORIAL ON ITEMS 45-49

The answers are: **45-A; 46-E; 47-D; 48-C; 49-C. Figure 1.7** is an electron micrograph of a **plasma cell**. Plasma cells differentiate from B-cells after appropriate antigenic stimulation and interaction with antigen presenting macrophages and helper T-cells. Plasma cells are highly differentiated cells dedicated to the synthesis and secretion of antibodies (**immunoglobulins**). Upon antigenic stimulation, the heterochromatinized nucleus of the B-lymphocyte decondenses to form a plasma cell nucleus with peripheral **heterochromatin** (B) and **euchromatin** (C). The **nucleolus** (D) contains the DNA sequences for the synthesis of ribosomal RNA, the essential component of ribosomes. Ribosomes bind to the endoplasmic reticulum to form the **rough endoplasmic reticulum** (A), the location where immunoglobulin mRNA is translated into the nascent polypeptide chains for immunoglobulin. Once synthesized, immunoglobulins are transported into the cisternae of the rough endoplasmic reticulum and then make their way out of the cell. **Mitochondria** (E) contain the enzymes for oxidative phosphorylation and electron transport crucial to the synthesis of ATP. Many of the anabolic functions of plasma cells are dependent on the energy-rich ATP produced in mitochondria.

ANSWERS AND TUTORIAL ON ITEMS 50-52

The answers are: **50-C; 51-C; 52-E.** Vitamin C deficiency results in a disease called **scurvy**. This disease is especially common in alcoholics because of dietary deficiency. Rupture of capillaries leads to follicular and gingival hemorrhages. Wound healing and fracture repair are also unusually slow in scorbutic patients. The granulation tissue at poorly healed wounds would have many **fibroblasts**, a cell type primarily involved in collagen biosynthesis. Vitamin C is an essential co-factor in enzymatic reactions catalyzing the hydroxylation of prolyl and lysyl residues of collagen. Procollagen molecules without hydroxyproline residues have significant instability in their triple helices and are therefore more susceptible to degradation. In addition, extracellular collagen molecules have few hydroxylysine residues. Their poor cross-linkage renders them more susceptible to **turnover**. Also, fibroblasts secrete collagen more slowly in the vitamin C deficient state. Bone growth and fracture repair are also abnormal in scurvy.

Items 53-56

Examine the scanning electron micrograph of a fractured specimen of liver tissue in **Figure 1.8** below. Match the labeled structure in the micrograph with the **MOST** appropriate microscopic anatomical or functional description of the labeled structure. Answers may be used once, more than once, or not at all.

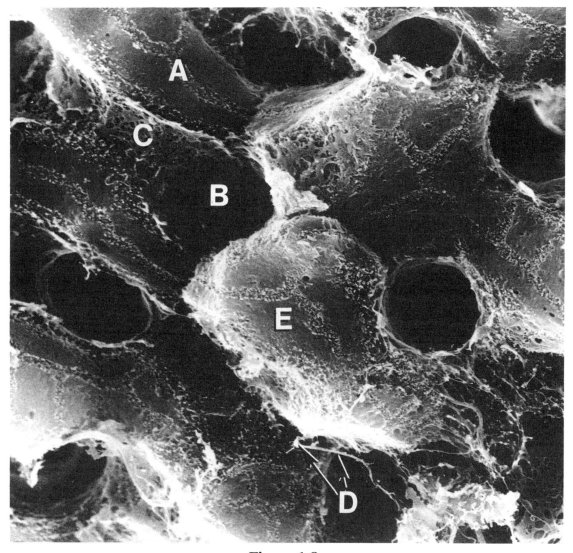

Figure 1.8

53. This structure receives blood from branches of the portal vein in the portal triads.

54. Liver parenchymal cells are joined by tight junctions at this structure to produce a blood-bile barrier.

55. This cell type is involved in synthesis of serum albumin and detoxification.

56. These endothelial cells form fenestrated and discontinuous capillaries.

ANSWERS AND TUTORIAL ON ITEMS 53-56

The answers are: **53-B; 54-A; 55-E; 56-C**. **Figure 1.8** is a scanning electron micrograph of fractured liver tissue. It consists numerous **liver parenchymal cells** (E) held together by delicate **collagen fibers** (D). Liver parenchymal cells are the main, functional, organ-specific cell type of the liver. They are involved in serum protein synthesis, metabolism of lipids and bile salts, and detoxification of drugs. Individual liver parenchymal cells are joined together by tight junctions on surfaces facing the **bile canaliculi** (A). These minute channels convey bile toward the portal canal where they join with hepatic ducts. Cords of liver parenchymal cells are surrounded by **sinusoids** (B) which convey blood from the portal triads to the central vein of a liver lobule. The **endothelial cells** (C) lining these sinusoids are arranged in a fenestrated and discontinuous layer and have some phagocytic capacity.

Items 57-59

For each organelle of the **placental syncytiotrophoblast**, select the **MOST** appropriate associated cellular function. Answers may be used once, more than once, or not at all.

(A) Rough endoplasmic reticulum
(B) Smooth endoplasmic reticulum
(C) Golgi apparatus
(D) Nuclear envelope
(E) Microvillus

57. Organelle that is involved in the final glycosylation of chorionic gonadotrophin.

58. Organelle that is involved in the synthesis of polypeptide chains for placental lactogen.

59. Organelle that is involved in absorption of nutrients.

ANSWERS AND TUTORIAL ON ITEMS 57-59

The answers are: **57-C; 58-A; 59-E**. The **syncytiotrophoblast** is the boundary between the maternal blood in the intervillous space of the placenta and the underlying fetal tissue of the placenta. The syncytiotrophoblast is formed by the proliferation and fusion of underlying **cytotrophoblasts** and is therefore a true syncytium. It has a complex ultrastructure that reflects the many different functions carried out in this syncytial epithelial layer. For example, the syncytiotrophoblast is the site of synthesis of **human chorionic gonadotrophin** (hCG), a glycoprotein hormone involved in maintaining the pregnant state of the female reproductive system during pregnancy. The polypeptides of hCG are synthesized in the **rough endoplasmic reticulum** (A) along with human placental lactogen and are glycosylated largely in the **Golgi apparatus** (C). Steroid biosynthesis probably occurs in part on the membranes of the rough endoplasmic reticulum. It should be noted that the smooth endoplasmic reticulum (B) is very poorly represented in the syncytiotrophoblast and therefore can not play a role in steroidogenesis. The **nuclear envelope** (D) is a double unit membrane with octagonal pores. It serves as the boundary between the nucleus and the cytoplasm. Microvilli are prominent on the apical border of the syncytiotrophoblast. Here, like in all other apical brush borders, the microvilli mediate fluid, small molecule and large molecule transport across the placenta. Inorganic ions, sugars and amino acids are actively transported across the placenta through the microvilli. Maternal immunoglobulins are engulfed functionally intact by pinocytosis and transported in some of the membrane bound **cytoplasmic vesicles** (E) found everywhere in the syncytiotrophoblast.

For each variety of epithelium, select the **MOST** appropriate associated anatomical location where this type of epithelium is found in the human body. Answers may be used once, more than once, or not at all.

       (A)   Simple squamous epithelium
       (B)   Simple cuboidal epithelium
       (C)   Simple columnar epithelium
       (D)   Pseudostratified columnar epithelium
       (E)   Stratified squamous epithelium, unkeratinized
       (F)   Stratified squamous epithelium, keratinized
       (G)   Stratified columnar epithelium
       (H)   Transitional epithelium

60.   Tracheal mucosa

61.   Visceral pleura

62.   Proximal convoluted tubule

63.   Epidermis

64.   Duodenal mucosa

ANSWERS AND TUTORIAL ON ITEMS 60-64

The answers are: **60-D; 61-A; 62-B; 63-E; 64-C**. **Simple squamous epithelium** (A) consists of a single layer of flattened epithelial cells. It is found at the lumen of all blood vessels (endothelium) and lining all serous cavities including the pleural cavities, pericardial cavity and peritoneal cavity (mesothelium). In all of these locations, the apical epithelial surface faces the lumen and prevents adhesion to maintain a patent lumen. In serous cavities, mesothelium secretes serous fluids and prevents adhesion of the visceral layer (on the organ) to the parietal layer (on the body wall). **Simple cuboidal epithelium** (B) consists of a single layer of cells that are equal in height and width. Simple cuboidal epithelium is found in proximal convoluted tubules, distal convoluted tubules and in the thyroid follicular epithelium. **Simple columnar epithelium** (C) consists of a single layer of cells that are taller than they are wide. This type of epithelium is present in the gastric and intestinal epithelium. Simple columnar epithelial cells often have a microvillous brush border that is involved in absorption of luminal contents. **Pseudostratified columnar epithelium** (D) consists of tall columnar epithelial cells that stretch all the way from the apex to the base of the epithelium and a variable population of cells resting on the basement membrane and reaching only part of the way up to the epithelial apex. It is found in the trachea, bronchi and large bronchioles of the respiratory system (where the tall columnar cells are ciliated) and is also widely distributed in the male reproductive system, e.g., in the epididymis, ductus deferens, prostate gland, and seminal vesicles. **Stratified squamous epithelium** is multilayered with flattened apical epithelial cells. It is found in the epidermis of the skin where it is keratinized (F) and in the esophagus and vagina where it is unkeratinized (E). Stratified squamous epithelium is specialized to resist abrasion. Stratified columnar epithelium (G) is multilayer with columnar apical cells. It is found in the penile urethra. **Transitional epithelium** (H) is multilayer with rounded, pillowy apical cells. It is restricted to the renal pelves, renal calyces, ureters, urinary bladder, and upper prostatic urethra in the male.

Items 65-73

For each variety of connective tissue, select the **MOST** appropriate associated anatomical location where this type of connective tissue is found in the human body. Answers may be used once, more than once, or not at all.

(A)   Loose irregular connective tissue
(B)   Dense irregular connective tissue
(C)   Dense regular connective tissue
(D)   Hyaline cartilage
(E)   Elastic cartilage
(F)   Fibrocartilage
(G)   Adipose tissue
(H)   Bone
(I)   Blood
(J)   Reticular connective tissue
(K)   Mucous connective tissue

65.   Forms the stroma of bone marrow.

66.   The articular surfaces of the humerus.

67.   The Achilles tendon.

68.   The auricle of the external ear.

69.   The reticular portion of the dermis.

70.   The lamina propria of the duodenum.

71.   Prominent packing material around kidneys and eyeball.

72.   Present in the umbilical cord as Wharton's jelly.

73.   Major constituent of annulus fibrosus.

ANSWERS AND TUTORIAL ON ITEMS 65-73

The answers are: **65-J; 66-D; 67-C; 68-E; 69-B; 70-A; 71-G; 72-K; 73-F. Loose irregular connective tissue** (A) consists of many cells and a few randomly arranged fibers. It often contains resident cells (fibroblasts) and immigrant cells such as neutrophils, macrophages and plasma cells. It forms the mucosal connective tissue (lamina propria) of the duodenum and all other moist visceral organs.

Dense irregular connective tissue (B) consists of a few cells and many densely packed fibers randomly arranged. It is most abundant in the deeper reticular layer of the dermis, the connective tissue of the skin.

Dense regular connective tissue (C) consists of a few cells and many densely packed fibers regularly arranged. The tendons are classical examples of dense regular connective tissue. Cartilage is a kind of specialized connective tissue along with bone, bone marrow, blood, reticular tissue and adipose tissue.

Hyaline cartilage (D) is abundant in the laryngeal and tracheal cartilages. It is also abundant in developing bones of the appendicular skeleton. Remnants of the cartilaginous models persist at the articular surfaces of long bones.

Elastic cartilage (E) is quite similar to hyaline cartilage histologically but it contains many elastic fibers. It is found in the epiglottis, around the auditory tube, in laryngeal cartilages and in the auricle (pinna) of the external ear.

Fibrocartilage (F) closely resembles dense regular connective tissue and intergrades with it where ligaments insert into bones. Unlike dense connective tissue, it contains chondrocytes surrounded by a small domain of metachromatic extracellular matrix. The intervertebral discs contain a tough outer capsule called the **nucleus pulposus** which consists of fibrocartilage.

Adipose tissue (G) is widely distributed throughout the body and is especially abundant in the hypodermis and the mesenteries. It serves as a store of excess lipids. Adipose tissue is also an important anatomical packing material around the kidneys and eyeball.

Bone (H) is a mineralized connective tissue. Its extracellular matrix contains predominantly type I collagen, glycosaminoglycans such as hyaluronic acid, keratan sulfate, and chondroitin sulfate, and hydroxyapatite ($Ca_{10}[PO_4]_6[OH]_2$)

Blood (I) is also a kind of connective tissue. Its cells are numerous, including erythrocytes and leucocytes. Its amorphous ground substance is the large number of proteins and glycoproteins (e.g., albumin and fibronectin) in the plasma. It also contains (potential) fibers in fibrinogen that become actual fibers when blot clots.

Reticular connective tissue (J) is a variety of loose connective tissue which contains fibers of type III collagen (reticular fibers). It also contains fibroblasts and macrophages. Reticular connective tissue forms the stroma of bone marrow, lymph nodes, the spleen, and the thymus.

Mucous connective tissue (K) has a peculiar abundance of amorphous ground substance rich in hyaluronic acid. Scattered collagen and reticular fibers are also present. In addition, the cell are mainly fibroblasts with a few macrophages. It is widespread in the early embryo and is the main connective tissue of the umbilical cord (**Wharton's jelly**) where its unusual physical properties prevent compression of umbilical blood vessels.

Items 74-79

For each variety of connective tissue protein, select the **MOST** appropriate associated anatomical or functional description of this molecule. Answers may be used once, more than once, or not at all.

(A)   Fibrillin
(B)   Elastin
(C)   Fibronectin
(D)   Type I Collagen
(E)   Type II collagen
(F)   Type III collagen
(G)   Type IV collagen
(H)   Thrombospondin
(I)   Laminin
(J)   Integrin

74.   The predominant fibrous protein of bone extracellular matrix.

75.   An adhesive glycoprotein, abundant in the extracellular matrix and blood plasma. Binds avidly to collagen and the cell surface via integrin.

76.   The most abundant constituent of the granules in platelets. Its release is involved in clot formation.

77.   This glycoprotein is a cruciform macromolecule abundant in the basement membrane.

78.   This transmembrane protein binds cells and extracellular matrix components via its extracellular domain and links to the cytoskeleton via its intracellular domain.

79.   Defects in this extracellular matrix protein are thought to be responsible for Marfan's syndrome.

The answers are: **74-D; 75-C; 76-H; 77-I; 78-J; 79-A**. **Fibrillin** (A) is a 350,000 MW unsulfated glycoprotein which is assembled into 9 nm microfibrils. These microfibrils are often associated with elastic fibers [which are rich in **elastin** (B)] and the basement membrane. Deficiencies of fibrillin result in Marfan's syndrome. Patients with **Marfan's syndrome** are usually tall and lanky. Defects in the wall of large blood vessels can often lead to fatal aneurysms.

   Fibronectin (C) is a 440,000 MW glycoprotein consisting of two polypeptide chains bound by -S-S- bridges. It has several different functional domains that interact strongly with and facilitate binding to collagen fibers, fibrin, cells, and extracellular matrix glycosaminoglycans. Cellular fibronectin is an important adhesive glycoprotein for many connective tissues. Plasma fibronectin is an essential element of the clotting cascade. It binds platelets to fibrin.

   Collagen is the most abundant protein in the body. Collagen is synthesized by many connective tissue cells. It forms fibrillar or amorphous masses, depending upon the specific type of collagen. Tropocollagen is a large linear macromolecule consisting of three intertwined α-helices. Larger masses of collagen, e.g., fibrils, are formed by side-to-side and end-to-end association of tropocollagen molecules and covalent cross-linking. **Type I Collagen** (D) is the most ubiquitous form of collagen, occurring in bones, tendons, the dermis, fascia, and the capsules around many visceral organs. **Type II collagen** (E) is abundant in hyaline cartilage, the nucleus pulposus of the intervertebral discs, and the vitreous body of the eye. **Type III collagen** (F) is abundant in the reticular fibers that lend support to the lamina propria, tunica media of blood vessels, and stroma of the liver, spleen, lymph nodes, thymus, kidney, and uterus. **Type IV collagen** (G) forms minute fibrils that are an essential constituent of the basement membrane, along with laminin and heparan sulfate proteoglycan

   Thrombospondin (H) is a 450,000 MW adhesive glycoprotein. It is the most abundant component of the granules in platelets. During clotting, these granules discharge, releasing thrombospondin which binds platelets to fibrinogen. It is also present in many connective tissues where its functional role is unclear.

   Laminin (I) is an approximately 1,000,000 MW glycoprotein composed of subunits assembled into a cruciform macromolecule. It is abundant in the basement membranes underlying epithelial cells and the basement membrane-like sheaths surrounding muscle cells. It has separate functional domains that recognize cell surfaces, type IV collagen, and heparan sulfate proteoglycan.

   Integrin (J) is a transmembrane protein that serves both as a receptor for several different extracellular matrix components and as an anchoring site for actin-rich microfilaments of the cytoskeleton. It consists of an α and β subunit. There are many varieties of both kind of subunit and they can be recombined in many different ways, conveying ligand specificity to the different kinds of integrins that exist.

Items 80-85

For each variety of connective tissue cell, select the **MOST** appropriate associated anatomical or functional description of this type of specialized connective tissue cell found in the human body. Answers may be used once, more than once, or not at all.

(A) Mesenchymal fibroblast
(B) Chondroblast
(C) Osteoblast
(D) Chondrocyte
(E) Osteocyte
(F) Mast cells
(G) Macrophage

80. This deep periosteal cell can differentiate into a type I collagen-secreting cell.

81. This perichondrial cell can differentiate into a type II collagen-secreting cell.

82. This cell responds to parathormone by osteolysis.

83. This cell type aggregates to form centers of chondrification in embryonic limb buds.

84. This cell is capable of mitotic division when surrounded by type II collagen and cartilage-specific proteoglycan.

85. This cell contains numerous metachromatic granules in its cytoplasm.

32

ANSWERS AND TUTORIAL ON ITEMS 80-85

The answers are: **80-C; 81-B; 82-E; 83-A; 84-D; 85-F. Mesenchymal fibroblasts** (A) are found in space-filling loose connective tissue in many embryonic locations including the developing limb buds. Here, they aggregate into centers of chondrification and then differentiate into chondroblasts and chondrocytes in cartilaginous models of bone.

Chondroblasts (B) are found in the inner layers of the perichondrium and are capable of differentiating into **chondrocytes** (D), mature cells of cartilage that are surrounded by type II collagen and cartilage-specific proteoglycan.

Osteoblasts (C) are found in the inner layers of the periosteum and all along the endosteum of bone. They secrete type I collagen and other matrix components that subsequently become calcified. Once osteoblasts have become entrapped in secreted calcified extracellular matrix, they are known as **osteocytes** (E). Osteocytes can both deposit calcium into new matrix under the influence of calcitonin or remove it from old matrix under the influence of parathormone. Osteocytes are the cells of mature bone. They have large numbers of cellular processes radiating from their surfaces. These processes interconnect individual osteocytes into extended networks via gap junctions. These osteocyte processes residue within minute canaliculi.

Mast cells (F) contain numerous metachromatic cytoplasmic granules rich in the anticoagulant heparin and histamine which increases capillary permeability. Mast cells have IgE bound to the surfaces. In allergic individuals, re-exposure to an antigen leads to degranulation of mast cells and inflammation. In severe cases, anaphylaxis occurs. The mast cells become explosively degranulated, leading to systemic increases in capillary permeability and potentially fatal decrease in blood pressure.

Macrophages (G) are the dedicated specific phagocytes of the body. They are derived from bone marrow. They have immunoglobulin and complement receptors on their cell surfaces. Monocytes are a reserve of undifferentiated macrophages in the blood and can quickly extravasate and differentiate into macrophages when and where needed. Opsonized bacteria are readily engulfed and destroyed by macrophages. Macrophages are also crucial for presenting antigen to lymphocytes in immune responses. The mononuclear phagocyte system includes all of the bone marrow-derived, dedicated phagocytes: histiocytes, alveolar macrophages, macrophages of the immune organs, Kupffer cells, microglia, osteoclasts, and Langerhans cells (of skin)

Examine the transmission electron micrograph of skeletal muscle in **Figure 1.9** below. Match the labeled structure in the micrograph with the **MOST** appropriate description of its microscopic anatomy or physiological role. Answers may be used once, more than once, or not at all.

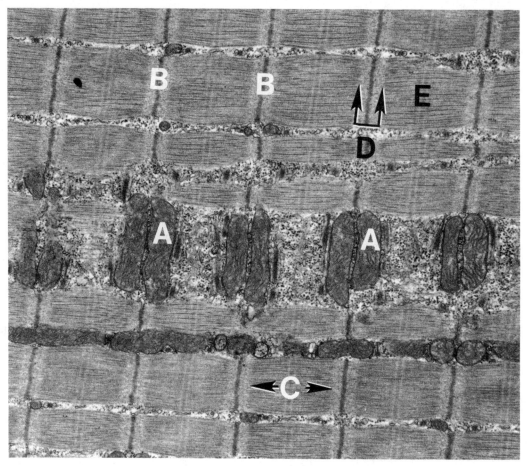

Figure 1.9

86. These structures define the ends of individual sarcomeres. They are regions rich in α-actinin.

87. These structures are regions of overlap between actin-rich thin filaments and myosin-rich thick filaments.

88. These structures produce ATP for muscle contraction.

89.   These structures are regions rich in actin-containing thin filaments where there is no overlap between thin and thick filaments.

90.   These structures are regions rich in myosin-containing thick filaments where there is no overlap between thick and thin filaments.

ANSWERS AND TUTORIAL ON ITEMS 86-90

The answers are: **86-B; 87-C; 88-A; 89-D; 90-E. Figure 1.9** is a high power transmission electron micrograph of skeletal muscle. Skeletal muscle fibers contain many myofibrils, each consisting of many **sarcomeres**. Each sarcomere is formed by a regular array of **thick** (myosin-rich) and **thin** (actin-rich) **filaments**. Myofibrils are composed of many sarcomeres. Individual sarcomeres extend from **Z line** (B) to Z line. Sarcomeres have central **A bands** (C) where there is extensive overlap between thin, actin-rich filaments and thick, myosin-rich filaments. When a muscle fiber (cell) contracts, the width of the **I bands** (D) and **H bands** (E) decreases because the thin and thick filaments increase their overlapping due to sliding of thin filaments past thick filaments. The H bands are regions of no overlap between thin and thick filaments. H bands contain no thin filaments. The length of the A bands remains constant during muscle contraction. During muscle contraction, the I bands and H bands decrease in length and the Z lines move closer together, leading to a shortening of the sarcomere. When many sarcomeres shorten, the entire muscle cell shortens. Muscle contraction is driven by the energy rich compound ATP which is produced in **mitochondria** (A).

Contractile force in muscle is generated by a change in the position of **actin and myosin**, which is regulated by intracellular **calcium** concentration. Energy for muscle contraction is derived from the hydrolysis of **ATP**. Under appropriate conditions, the actin-myosin complex has ATPase activity. Release of energy from ATP hydrolysis causes conformational changes in the muscle proteins resulting in useful movement. A sarcomere has a variable total length depending on the contractile status of the cell. When a muscle contracts, thick and thin filaments slide past one another. During a contraction and relaxation cycle, calcium concentration around the myofibrils increases suddenly. This causes a conformational change in the **troponin** molecule, which exposes the **S-1** (cross-bridge) binding site of actin, and a myosin-actin complex forms. Another conformational change occurs, and the S-1 fragment, still in association with the actin-containing thin filament, swings like an oar in an oarlock and causes the thin filament to slide relative to the thick filament. When this occurs at millions of cross-bridges, the entire sarcomere is shortened. The calcium concentration falls rapidly, following hydrolysis of ATP and the swinging of cross-bridges. The drop in calcium severs the association between actin and myosin and the contraction stops. ATP is hydrolysed to adenosine diphosphate (ADP), which subsequently is phosphorylated to form ATP. The hydrolysis and regeneration of ATP in muscle contraction explains the plethora of **mitochondria** in skeletal and cardiac muscle.

Items 91-93

Examine the transmission electron micrograph in **Figure 1.10** below and then choose the **MOST** appropriate answer. Answers may be used once, more than once, or not at all.

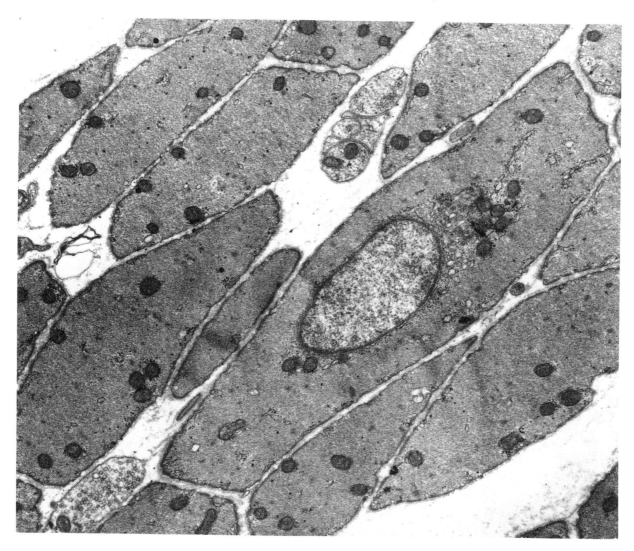

Figure 1.10

91. The predominant cell type in this electron micrograph is

   (A)   fibroblast
   (B)   chondrocyte
   (C)   cardiac muscle cell
   (D)   smooth muscle cell
   (E)   adipocyte

92.   This cell type is most abundant in

    (A)   a tendon
    (B)   hyaline cartilage
    (C)   the cardiac ventricular walls
    (D)   the wall of the urinary bladder
    (E)   white fat

93.   Which constituent would be most abundant in the cytoplasm of these cells?

    (A)   actin
    (B)   type I collagen
    (C)   type II collagen
    (D)   cholesterol esters
    (E)   cartilage proteoglycan

ANSWERS AND TUTORIAL ON ITEMS 91-93

The answers are: **91-D; 92-D; 93-A. Figure 1.10** is a low power electron micrograph of smooth muscle cells in the wall of the **urinary bladder**. Moist, hollow visceral organs including the urinary bladder have a luminal mucosa which consists of epithelium and lamina propria, a submucosa, a muscularis externa and an adventitial layer. When the adventitial layer is coated by a simple squamous epithelium (mesothelium), it is called the serosa. The muscularis externa in these visceral organs is rich in **smooth muscle cells**. These cells have a single nucleus per cell like cardiac muscle cells but lack the striations of cardiac muscle cells. Skeletal muscle cells have striations like cardiac muscle cells but have larger cells containing many nuclei (derived from many separate myoblasts) enclosed within a single plasma membrane (called the sarcolemma in the case of muscle cells). Smooth muscle cells have actin, myosin, troponin and tropomyosin but these contractile proteins are not arranged in well-organized sarcomeres. This is the reason that smooth muscle cells are not striated like skeletal muscle and cardiac muscle cells. The contractions of smooth muscle cells in the muscularis externa of hollow visceral organs regulates the diameter of the lumen. In the case of the urinary bladder, contraction of smooth muscle cells occurs when the full bladder contracts and empties urine into the urethra.

Items 94-97

Examine the scanning electron micrograph of fractured tissue in **Figure 1.11** below and then choose the **BEST** response to the items.

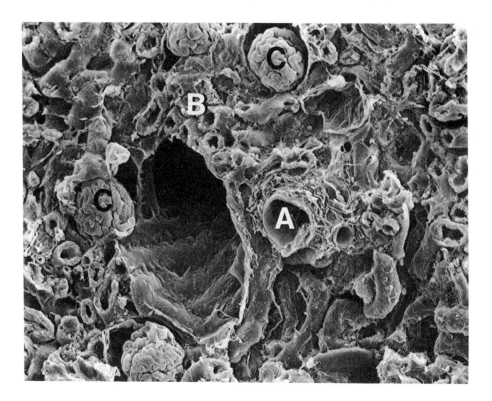

Figure 1.11

94. Structure A contains which of the following fluids?

   (A) blood
   (B) lymph
   (C) bile
   (D) glomerular filtrate
   (E) cerebrospinal fluid

95. Structure B has which of the following physiological roles?

   (A) modification of glomerular filtrate
   (B) nutrient and waste transport
   (C) O_2 and CO_2 transport
   (D) bile transport
   (E) chylomicron transport

96.   Structure C has which of the following physiological roles?

(A)   nutrient absorption
(B)   hormone synthesis
(C)   blood filtration to remove nitrogenous wastes
(D)   gas transport
(E)   lymphocyte transport

97.   This morphological arrangement is found in the

(A)   adrenal cortex
(B)   liver parenchyma
(C)   brain parenchyma
(D)   thymic cortex
(E)   renal cortex

ANSWERS AND TUTORIAL ON ITEMS 94-97

The answers are: **94-A; 95-A; 96-C; 97-E. Figure 1.11** is a low power scanning electron micrograph of the **renal cortex**. The cortical portion of the kidneys consists of large numbers of **blood vessels** (A), **renal corpuscles** (C) and **tubules** (B). Large branches of the renal arteries carry blood rich in nitrogenous wastes into the afferent arterioles which supply a glomerular capillary tuft in the renal corpuscles. The glomerular capillary tuft resides in a deep invagination of Bowman's capsule, the other portion of the renal corpuscle. Bowman's capsule has a visceral epithelial layer consisting of podocytes and a parietal layer consisting of simple squamous epithelial cells that are continuous with the cuboidal epithelial cells of the proximal convoluted tubule. The glomerular blood filtrate crosses the glomerular basement membrane, passes between the foot processes of **podocytes** and enters the urinary space of the renal corpuscle. The urinary pole of Bowman's capsule conveys dilute urine into the proximal convoluted tubules where the complex process of recovery of proteins and salts from the blood filtrate begins.

As the filtrate passes through the proximal convoluted tubules, loop of Henle, distal convoluted tubules and collecting tubules, the blood filtrate is modified further by recovery of most of the protein that crosses the glomerular basement membrane and by changes in salt and urea concentrations to produce urine.

Examine the scanning electron micrograph in **Figure 1.12** below and then choose the **MOST** correct answer. Answers may be used once, more than once, or not at all.

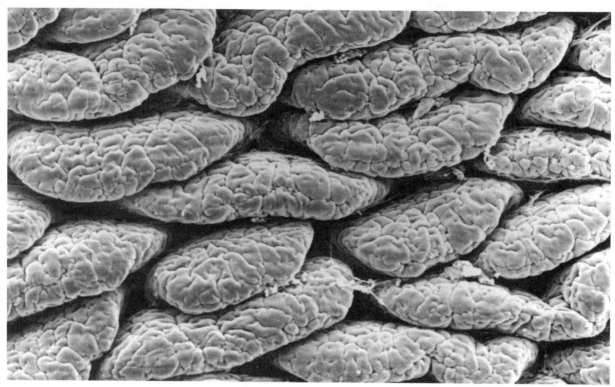

Figure 1.12

98.   These structures have which major physiological function?

    (A)   taste perception
    (B)   nutrient absorption
    (C)   bile concentration
    (D)   gamete transport
    (E)   blood transport

99.   These structures are characteristic of the mucosal surface of which organ?

    (A)   stomach
    (B)   jejunum
    (C)   uterine tube
    (D)   tongue
    (E)   gall bladder

100. The mucosal epithelium here consists of

    (A)   ciliated and secretory cells
    (B)   ciliated cells only
    (C)   absorptive cells and goblet cells
    (D)   a pseudostratified ciliated columnar epithelium with goblet cells
    (E)   transitional epithelium

ANSWERS AND TUTORIAL ON ITEMS 98-100

The answers are: **98-B; 99-B; 100-C**. **Figure 1.12** is a scanning electron micrograph of the mucosal surface of the **jejunum**, the second longest component of the small intestine. While some digestion and nutrient absorption occurs in the stomach, most of the digestion and nutrient absorption occurs in the small intestine. The mucosa of the jejunum has a plethora of **villi**. Jejunal villi are long flat structures covered by a simple columnar epithelium consisting of many tall, thin, columnar absorptive cells with an apical microvillous brush border. These cells are primarily responsible for absorption of digested nutrients from the lumen of the small intestine. In addition, the jejunal mucosal epithelium has goblet cells interspersed between columnar absorptive cells. Goblet cells secrete a thick coat of mucus that protects the jejunal mucosa from digestion.

Items 101-104

Examine the high power transmission electron micrograph of the junctions between three liver parenchymal cells in **Figure 1.13** below and then choose the **MOST** correct answer. Answers may be used once, more than once, or not at all.

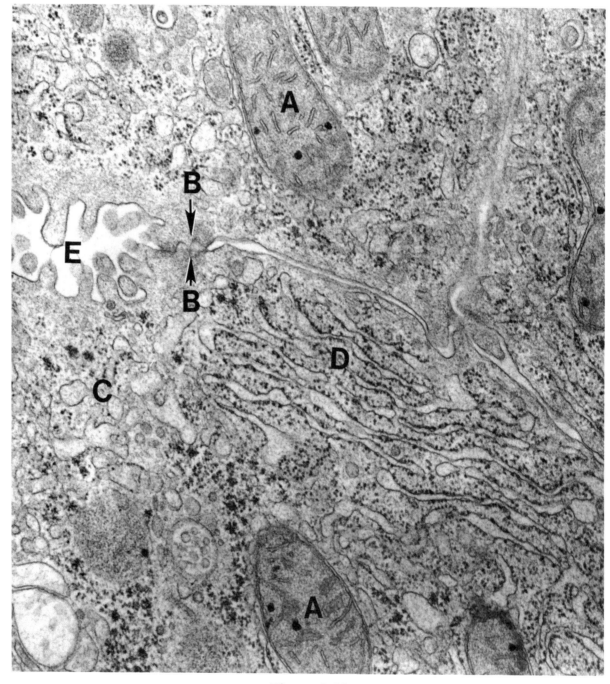

Figure 1.13

101. This structure contains enzymes for the electron transport chain and oxidative phosphorylation.

102. This structure forms a tight anatomical junction which serves as the blood-bile barrier.

103. This structure is involved in the initial stages of the synthesis of serum albumin.

104. This structure conveys bile toward the hepatic ducts.

ANSWERS AND TUTORIAL ON ITEMS 101-104

The answers are: **101-A; 102-B; 103-D; 104-E. Figure 1.13** is a high power transmission electron micrograph of a part of three liver parenchymal cells. **Mitochondria** (A) have enzymes for the electron transport chain and oxidative phosphorylation. These enzymes are used to synthesize ATP. This energy rich compound is utilized for many of the anabolic processes occurring in the liver. For example, the liver is actively engaged in protein synthesis. The **rough endoplasmic reticulum** (D) is the site where mRNAs are translated into polypeptide chains. Bile constituents are conjugated in the **smooth endoplasmic reticulum** (C) and are secreted into the **bile canaliculi** (E) between parenchymal cells. **Tight junctions** (B) surround the bile canaliculi and prevent bile from leaking into the vascular spaces in the liver. Thus, these tight junctions represent the anatomical basis for the blood-bile barrier.

Examine this high power transmission electron micrograph in **Figure 1.14** below. It is an array of long hollow structures cut perpendicular to their long axis. The diameter of each hollow structure is 25 nm. Choose the **BEST** response.

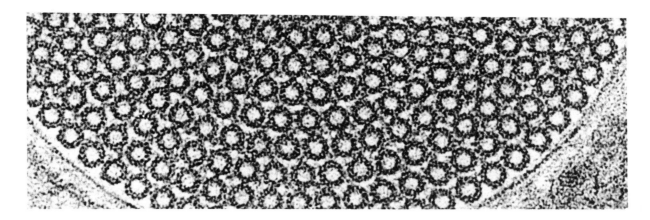

Figure 1.14

105.   Each individual circular structure is a(n)

     (A)   microfilament
     (B)   ciliary axoneme
     (C)   microtubule
     (D)   thick filament of muscle
     (E)   intermediate filament

106.   The most abundant protein found in these structures is

     (A)   tubulin
     (B)   actin
     (C)   keratin
     (D)   desmin
     (E)   myosin

107.   Which of the following proteins is present in abundance?

     (A)   actin
     (B)   vimentin
     (C)   microtubule associated proteins
     (D) α-actinin
     (E)   tropomyosin

108.   Which description is most appropriate for these structures?

(A)   The thick filaments are composed of aggregates of myosin molecules.
(B)   Dynein rich side-arms are involved in their movement.
(C)   They consist of globular actin molecules arranged in two intertwined helices with troponin and tropomyosin molecules arrayed along the helix.
(D)   They consist of 13 protofilaments composed of alternating α- and ß-tubulin subunits arranged like a string of beads.
(E)   They are abundant in the cores of microvilli.

ANSWERS AND TUTORIAL ON ITEMS 105-108

The answers are: **105-C; 106-A; 107-C; 108-D**. **Figure 1.14** is a high power transmission electron micrograph of an array of **microtubules** cut perpendicular to their long axis. Microtubules are long hollow structures with an outside diameter of 25 nm. They consist of 13 protofilaments. Each protofilament consists of alternating subunits of α- and ß-**tubulin**. Tubulins have similar molecular weights (55 kD) but are distinct due to subtle chemical differences. In addition to tubulin, microtubules have microtubule associated proteins that are involved in the interaction of microtubules with other cytoskeletal elements. Microtubules are important **cytoskeletal structures** that are involved in maintenance of cell morphology. They are also important constituents of cilia, flagella, centrioles and the mitotic spindle. Microtubules are important for moving entire cells as well as chromosomes within cells during mitosis.

Examine the high power transmission electron micrograph of cell surface projections in **Figure 1.15** below. These projections are cut perpendicular to their long axis. Match the **MOST** appropriate description of the functional role of the structure with the labeled structure in the electron micrograph.

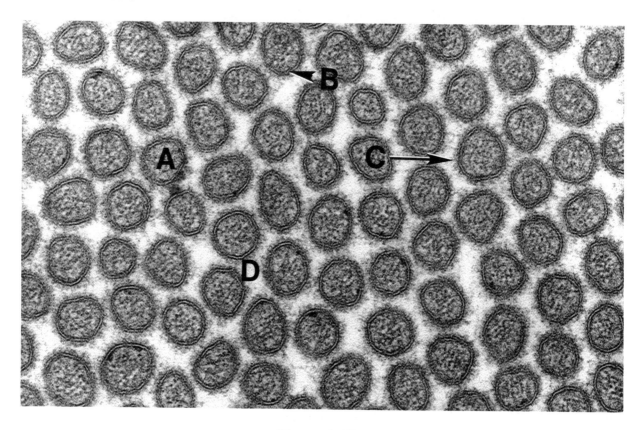

Figure 1.15

109. These structures are actin-rich microfilaments. They have a structural role.

110. These structures are a phospholipoprotein bilayer serving as a selective permeability barrier surrounding the entire cell.

111. This is a glycoprotein rich layer containing enzymatic activities for the hydrolysis of disaccharides.

112. These surface projections have which primary physiological function?

(A) movement of luminal contents
(B) transduction of mechanical into electrical energy
(C) transduction of chemical into electrical energy
(D) absorption of luminal contents
(E) gas exchange

ANSWERS AND TUTORIAL ON ITEMS 109-112

The answers are: **109-A; 110-B; 111-C; 112-D**. **Figure 1.15** is a high power transmission electron micrograph of sections cut perpendicular to the long axis of the **microvilli** in the jejunum of the small intestine. Microvilli are apical surface projections designed to increase the cell surface area. They are particularly well developed in areas where luminal contents are being absorbed, e.g., in the small and large intestine and proximal and distal convoluted tubules in the kidneys. Like all other cell surface projections, microvilli are covered by a phospholipoprotein bilayer of the **plasma membrane** (B). The cores of microvilli are filled with many **microfilaments** (A) with a diameter of 6 nm. These microfilaments are rich in actin and are involved in movement of microvilli.

The plasma membrane of intestinal microvilli has a thick **glycocalyx** (C) which consists of the glycoprotein rich extracellular domains of integral membrane proteins. This fuzzy coat on the outer leaflet of the plasma membrane consists of minute filaments, 2.5-5 nm in diameter. They often project 0.1 to 0.5 μm beyond the apical tips of microvilli into the **luminal space** (D) of the jejunum. The glycocalyx prevents digestive enzymes in the lumen of the small intestine from gaining access to epithelial cells. In addition, the glycocalyx contains digestive enzymes that complete the final steps in nutrient digestion.

Examine the light micrograph in **Figure 1.16** below and then choose the **MOST** appropriate labeled structure to match the functional role or morphological description of this structure. Answers may be used once, more than once, or not at all.

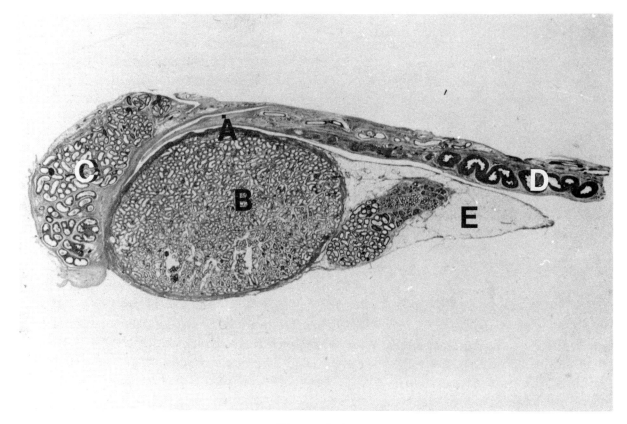

Figure 1.16

113. This structure has a pseudostratified epithelial lining and a thick coat of smooth muscle. It leads directly into the ejaculatory ducts.

114. This thick connective tissue capsule has septa that divide its enclosed tissue into lobules.

115. This structure is lined by a pseudostratified epithelium with long stereocilia. Spermatozoa undergo maturation here.

116. This structure contains both Sertoli cells and Leydig cells. Spermatogenesis occurs here.

ANSWERS AND TUTORIAL ON ITEMS 113-116

The answers are: **113-D; 114-A; 115-C; 116-B. Figure 1.16** is a low power light micrograph of a sagittal section through the **testis** (B), **tail of the epididymis** (C) and **ductus deferens** (D). The testis is encapsulated by a dense fibrous connective tissue capsule called the **tunica albuginea** (A). **Adipose tissue** (E) is associated with the head of the epididymis. Septa penetrate deep into the testis from the tunica albuginea and divide each testis into several hundred testicular lobules. Each lobule consists of many seminiferous tubules. Spermatogenesis, a process where proliferative spermatogonia differentiate into primary spermatocytes and eventually haploid spermatozoa, occurs in the seminiferous tubules of the testis. Meiosis begins in the primary spermatocyte, eventually resulting in the formation of millions of haploid spermatozoa.

The seminiferous tubules are surrounded by interstitial tissue rich in connective tissue fibroblasts, fenestrated capillaries and testosterone-secreting **Leydig cells**. Spermatogenesis and the secretory activities of the excurrent duct system of the testes are testosterone-dependent. The seminiferous tubules empty into the rete testis which in turn empties into the **efferent ductules**. The efferent ductules join the head of the epididymis, a long convoluted tube interconnecting the efferent ductules and the ductus deferens. The mucosal epithelium of the epididymis and ductus deferens are both pseudostratified columnar. Spermatozoa are thought to mature in the epididymis. They are conveyed through the ductus deferens into the prostate and out the penile urethra during ejaculation.

Items 117-120

For each cell of the immune system, select the **MOST** appropriate functional role in the immune response.

        (A)   Macrophage
        (B)   Helper T-cell
        (C)   Natural killer cell
        (D)   B-cell
        (E)   Plasma cell

117.   In conjunction with antigen-presenting and antibody producing cell, this cell is required for antibody synthesis.

118.   This cell is a bone marrow derivative involved in presentation of antigen to immunoglobulin producing cell.

119.   This cell has an abundant rough endoplasmic reticulum and a prominent nucleolus. It dedicated to immunoglobulin synthesis and secretion into the blood.

120.   This cell has a granular cytoplasm with azurophilic granules. It is a differentiated cell which represents the first line of defense against foreign cells.

ANSWERS AND TUTORIAL ON ITEMS 117-120

The answers are: **117-B; 118-A; 119-E; 120-C**. The immune system contains a diverse assortment of cells for defense against foreign antigens and foreign cells. In the humoral immune response, **B-cells** (D) differentiate into immunoglobulin secreting **plasma cells** (E). **Macrophages** (A) are derived from bone marrow and in conjunction with **helper T-cells** (B) must present foreign antigens to B-cells to control their differentiation into plasma cells. Once B-cells are stimulated to differentiate into plasma cells, their nucleus becomes less condensed, a nucleolus appears for synthesis of ribosomal RNA and the cytoplasmic compartment of the cell expands to accommodate an increase in rough endoplasmic reticulum and Golgi apparatus. The cytoplasmic machinery for immunoglobulin synthesis and secretion thus appears as a B-cell differentiates into a plasma cell. Our immune system also contains a population of **natural killer (NK) cells** (C). NK cells are highly differentiated cell types that serve as the first line of defense against foreign cells. They are cytolytic entities and can act directly on foreign cell types, thus destroying them rapidly. The formation of killer T-cells from small lymphocytes in response to foreign cells requires a delay, during which an abnormal tumor cell might proliferate more rapidly than the killer T-cells designed to combat the transformed cell. When a tumor arises, NK cells probably attack it first and limit the further development of tumor cells until a new cadre of killer T-cells forms a second line of defense against the malignant tumor cells. They are larger than lymphocytes (12-15 μm), have a lobulated nucleus and many cytoplasmic azurophilic granules.

For each organ of the immune system, select the **MOST** appropriate functional role in the immune response.

>   (A)   Lymph node
>   (B)   Spleen
>   (C)   Liver
>   (D)   Thymus
>   (E)   Bone marrow

121.   This organ is derived from pharyngeal pouches III and IV. It contains reticular epithelial cells and lymphocytes.

122.   This organ has a subcapsular sinus. Germinal centers appear in response to antigenic stimulation.

123.   This organ is responsible for immune surveillance of the blood and removal of effete erythrocytes from the systemic circulation.

124.   This organ is the first major hematopoietic organ in the embryo.

The labeled light micrographs in **Figure 1.17** below are taken from the deep (left) and superficial (right) portions of the fundic gastric pits. Choose the **MOST** appropriate description of the morphology or functional role of the labeled cell type. Answers may be used once, more than once, or not at all.

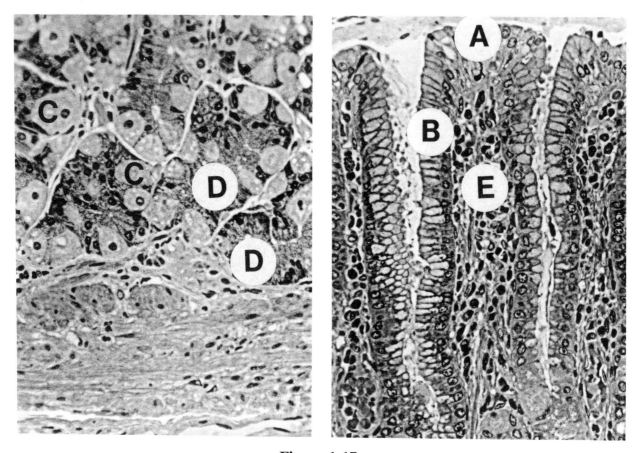

Figure 1.17

125. These cells are acidophilic, have an extensive apical canalicular system and have many mitochondria closely associated with the canaliculi.

126. These cells have a basophilic cytoplasm rich in rough endoplasmic reticulum. They secrete pepsinogen.

127. These mucous surface cells secrete a protective layer of mucus and form the most superficial cells of the gastric glands.

128.   These cells secrete gastric intrinsic factor.

129.   The secretion of these cells is sensitive to gastrin.

ANSWERS AND TUTORIAL ON ITEMS 121-124

The answers are: **121-D; 122-A; 123-B; 124-C. Lymph nodes** (A) are distributed widely throughout the body. They are especially abundant in the cervical, axillary and inguinal regions where they receive the lymphatic drainage of the head, upper extremities and lower extremities respectively. Lymph nodes receive lymph via peripheral afferent lymphatics. These vessels convey lymph into the subcapsular sinuses and then allow it to circulate slowly over germinal centers distributed throughout the cortex. Germinal centers contain macrophages, lymphocytes and plasma cells. After percolating past germinal centers, lymph drains into sinuses in the medullary portion of the node and exits via the efferent lymphatics in the hilus. The lymph nodes are responsible for the immune surveillance of the lymph.

The **spleen** (B) is located in the dorsal mesentery of the stomach. It consists of white pulp (periarterial lymphatic sheaths = PALS) and red pulp. The PALS contain germinal centers and are responsible for production of antibodies directed against blood-borne antigens. The red pulp consists of a complex network of sinusoids that entrap and destroy aged and damaged erythrocytes. The **liver** (C) is a relatively large organ in the embryo. It serves as the major hematopoietic organ after the yolk sac regresses and before the **bone marrow** (E) develops into the predominant site of hematopoiesis.

The **thymus** (D) is a lobulated organ consisting of reticular epithelial cells derived from the IIIrd and IVth pharyngeal pouches (endoderm) and large numbers of lymphocytes. The reticular epithelial cells secrete a protein called thymosin which is required for differentiation of T-cells. T-cells formed in the thymus then leave the organ and are dispersed widely throughout the blood, peripheral connective tissues, lymph nodes and spleen.

ANSWERS AND TUTORIAL ON ITEMS 125-129

The answers are: **125-C; 126-D; 127-A; 128-C; 129-C**. **Figure 1.17** is a light micrograph of the **gastric mucosa** which has many glandular pits throughout the fundic and corpic regions. These glands have several different kinds of epithelial cells. The most superficial portion of gastric glands contains **mucous surface cells** (A). These cells extend a short way into the upper portion of gastric glands but are soon replaced by **mucous neck cells** (B). Both cells are similar in their structure but secrete mucus with differing chemical properties. Their secretions coat the gastric mucosa and prevent its ulceration by the proteolytic enzymes inside the gastric lumen. Beneath the mucous neck cells, one encounters **parietal cells** (C) and **chief cells** (D). Parietal cells are more abundant in the upper portions of the gastric glands. They have a complex apical canalicular system that serves to increase their surface area. These cells also have a large number of acidophilic mitochondria closely associated with the canalicular system. Parietal cells secrete HCl and **gastric intrinsic factor**. Enteroendocrine cells known as **G cells** secrete **gastrin**, a polypeptide that stimulates HCl secretion from parietal cells. Gastric intrinsic factor is required for absorption of vitamin B_{12}. Chief cells are more abundant in the deepest portions of gastric glands. Chief cells have a fine structure that is appropriate for the synthesis and secretion of the main digestive enzyme of the stomach, **pepsinogen**. Thus, they have a basophilic cytoplasm with an abundance of rough endoplasmic reticulum, abundant mitochondria, a well developed Golgi apparatus and zymogen granules containing pepsinogen. Once secreted, pepsinogen is cleaved to pepsin, a form with proteolytic activity and a pH optimum around 2.0. The gastric mucosa also has a **lamina propria** (E) consisting of a loose areolar connective tissue rich in fibroblasts.

Items 130-133

Examine the labeled light micrograph in **Figure 1.18** below and then choose the **MOST** appropriate description of the morphology or functional role of the labeled structure. Answers may be used once, more than once, or not at all.

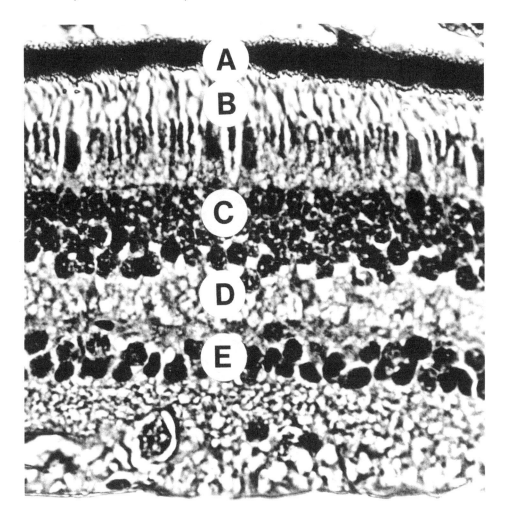

Figure 1.18

130. This structure contains the nuclei of bipolar cells, horizontal cells and amacrine cells.

131. This structure contains the nuclei of rods and cones.

132. This structure is rich in melanin. The apical surfaces of epithelial cells here phagocytose the apical portion of effete rod and cone outer segments.

133. This structure contains neuronal processes connecting rods and cones to bipolar cell.

ANSWERS AND TUTORIAL ON ITEMS 130-133

The answers are: **130-E; 131-C; 132-A; 133-D**. **Figure 1.18** is a photomicrograph of the photoreceptive portion of the **retina**. The innermost layer here consists of the **pigmented retina** (A). This is a simple cuboidal epithelium of melanin-containing pigmented cells. It functions to absorb stray light and also phagocytoses the apical portions of the **outer segments of the rods and cones** (B). The nuclei of the rods and cones are contained in the **outer nuclear layer** (C). Axons of these rods and cones project through the **outer plexiform layer** (D) and synapse with dendrites of bipolar cells, the nuclei of which are found in the **inner nuclear layer** (E) along with the nuclei of **Müller cells**, horizontal cells and amacrine cells. Müller cells are supportive, tall columnar cells that span much of the thickness of the neural retina. Horizontal cells integrate signals from multiple photoreceptors. **Amacrine cells** establish contacts between ganglion cells. Their function is poorly understood. Processes extending between the inner nuclear layer and the ganglion cell layer are found in the **inner plexiform layer**. Ganglion cells have their nuclei in the ganglion cell layer and project axons toward the optic nerve through the **optic nerve fiber layer**.

Examine the labeled light micrograph in **Figure 1.19** below and then choose the **MOST** appropriate description of the morphology or functional role of the labeled structure. Answers may be used once, more than once, or not at all.

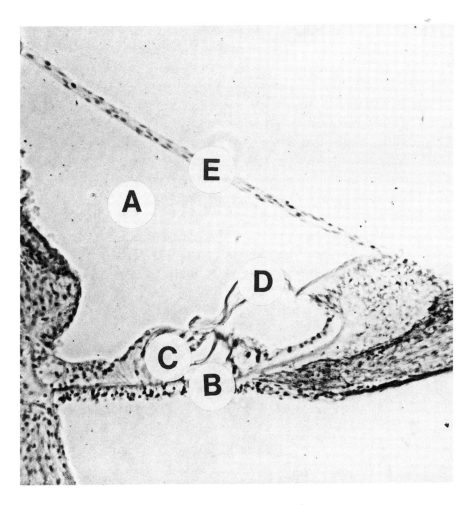

Figure 1.19

134. The apical surfaces of hair cells contact this structure.

135. This structure contains a blood filtrate which is produced in the stria vascularis and resorbed in the endolymphatic sac.

136. The apical projections from this structure are highly modified microvilli.

137. Basilar fibers are located in this structure.

ANSWERS AND TUTORIAL ON ITEMS 134-137

The answers are: **134-D; 135-A; 136-C; 137-B**. **Figure 1.19** is a light micrograph of the **organ of Corti**, the mechanoreceptor in the inner ear responsible for converting vibrations into electrical impulses for sound perception. The organ of Corti resides within an endolymph-filled cavity called the **cochlear duct** (scala media) (A). Endolymph is a blood filtrate secreted into the cochlear duct at the stria vascularis and resorbed in a diverticulum of the membranous labyrinth called the endolymphatic sac. The organ of Corti rests on the **basilar membrane** (B). Basilar fibers reside in the basilar membrane. Traveling waves of deflection are produced in the basilar membrane by vibrations in the oval window. These waves are damped out at different locations along the basilar membrane depending upon the frequency of the traveling waves, resulting in stimulation of different **hair cells** (C) depending upon the frequency of the sound. Hair cells have long apical microvilli that contact the relatively stationary **tectorial membrane** (D). When the basilar membrane moves the hair cells, their apical microvilli are deformed because they move with respect to the relatively fixed tectorial membrane. These deformations lead to the initiation of action potentials from hair cells. Subsequently, these action potentials are conducted into the brain where they are perceived as sounds. The **vestibular membrane** (E) is the boundary between the cochlear duct and the scala vestibuli. The basilar membrane is the boundary between the cochlear duct and the scala tympani. The scala vestibuli and the scala tympani are continuous with one another. Both are filled with perilymph.

Items 138-144

Examine the labeled diagram of a typical renal pyramid in **Figure 1.20** below and then choose the **BEST** anatomical or functional description of the labeled structures. Answers may be used once, more than once, or not at all.

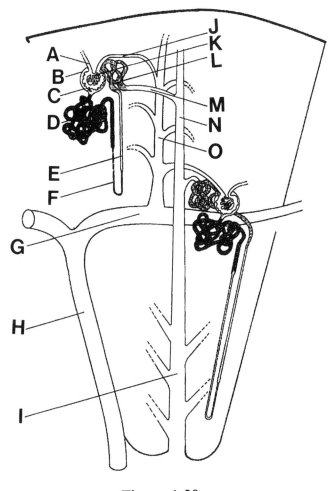

Figure 1.20

138. Juxtaglomerular cells in the wall of this structure secrete renin.

139. Macula densa cells in the wall of this structure sense ionic composition of glomerular filtrate. Part of the juxtaglomerular apparatus.

140.   Immediate upstream blood supply for glomerulus.

141.   Branches of this vessel form the vasa recta and capillaries around proximal and distal convoluted tubules. Note: vessel is shown but branches are not!

142.   The most prominent microvilli are found here. It is the site of most protein resorption from glomerular filtrate.

143.   This structure is lined by a simple squamous epithelium. It leads immediately into the proximal convoluted tubule.

144.   This structure conveys urine most directly into the distal convoluted tubules.

ANSWERS AND TUTORIAL ON ITEMS 138-144

The answers are: **138-J; 139-L; 140-J; 141-A; 142-D; 143-B; 144-E**. **Figure 1.20** is a diagram of the distribution of nephrons and their arterial blood supply in a single renal pyramid. Branches from the renal artery convey blood into the **interlobar artery** (H) which in turn leads to the **arcuate artery** (G) at the cortico-medullary junction. Branches from the arcuate artery, known at **interlobular artery** (O) course toward the superficial renal cortex, sending off **afferent arterioles** (J) which are the immediate afferent blood supply for renal **glomeruli** (K). The **efferent arteriole** (A) conducts blood away from the glomerulus and then supplies a complex anastomosing network of capillaries surrounding the proximal and distal convoluted tubules and forming **vasa recta** that parallel the loops of Henle (not shown in the diagram). These vessels then enter the venous drainage of the kidney (not shown in diagram). The **glomerular filtrate** passes through glomerular capillaries and enters **Bowman's space** (C). The visceral layer of Bowman's capsule consists of a unique population of **podocytes**, octopus-like cells which form part of the blood-urine barrier (along with the **glomerular basement membrane** and the **fenestrated** (without diaphragms) glomerular capillaries. The **parietal layer of Bowman's capsule** (B) consists of the simple squamous epithelium that is directly continuous with the **proximal convoluted tubule** (D) (PCT), the site of most water, nutrient, salt, and protein resorption from the glomerular filtrate. After passing through the PCT the glomerular filtrate passes through the **descending thick and thin limbs** (F) of the **loop of Henle** and enters the **ascending thin and thick limbs** (E) of the loop of Henle. From the loop of Henle, the glomerular filtrate passes into the **distal convoluted tubule** (L) (DCT), the **collecting tubule**

(M), **collecting duct** (N) and **papillary duct** (I). Papillary ducts (of Bellini) empty into the minor calyces at the **area cribrosa** of the renal papilla. From there urine, is conveyed into the major calyces, renal pelvis, ureters, urinary bladder, and then out of the body through the urethra.

The **juxtaglomerular apparatus** plays a crucial role in the regulation of the ionic composition of urine and blood. It also is an important regulator of blood pressure. It consists of three important components:

1) **Juxtaglomerular cells** which are modified smooth muscle cells in the wall of the **afferent arteriole** (J). These cells contain and secrete granules of the hydrolytic enzyme **renin**. When blood pressure falls, renin is secreted. Renin hydrolyses the blood protein **angiotensinogen** into a decapeptide **angiotensin I** which is in turn hydrolysed by **angiotensin converting enzyme** (ACE) to **angiotensin II**, an octapeptide that is an extremely potent vasoconstrictor. An increase in angiotensin II causes an increase in blood pressure and renin secretion is inhibited. ACE inhibitors such as **captopril** reduce the production of angiotensin II and thus lower blood pressure.

2) **Macula densa cells** which are found in the wall of the DCT (L) as it meets the vascular pole of the renal corpuscle. These tall columnar epithelial cells probably represent sensory elements that monitor the osmotic conditions in the distal convoluted tubule.

3) **Extraglomerular mesangial cells** (also called lacis cells or Goormaghtigh cells) are found in the extraglomerular interstitium adjacent to glomerular capillary cells at the vascular pole of the renal corpuscle. These cells contact glomerular capillary endothelial cells, juxtaglomerular cells, and the macula densa by way of gap junctions. These cells probably coordinate activities of the other two components of the juxtaglomerular apparatus by unknown means.

CHAPTER II
EMBRYOLOGY

Items 145-154

Examine the photomicrograph in **Figure 2.1** below and then match the labeled structure with the **MOST** appropriate description of its functional role in gametogenesis in the items that follow. Answers may be used once, more than once, or not at all.

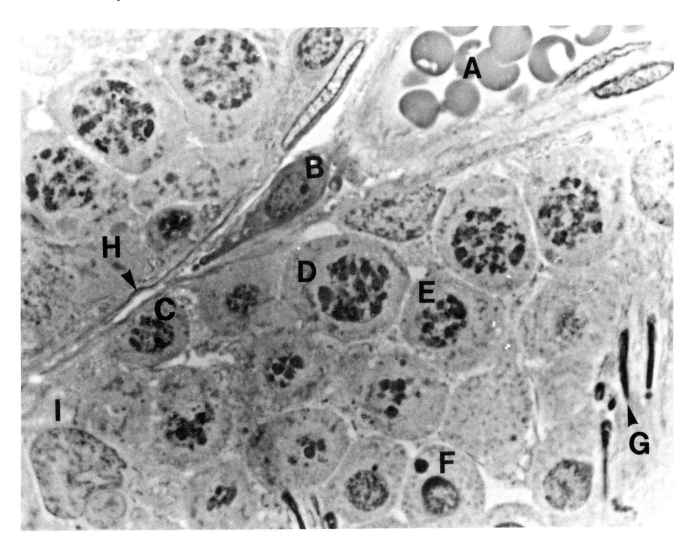

Figure 2.1

A - capillary
B - Leydig cell
C - spermatogonia (2n)
D - 1° spermatocyte (4n)
E - 2° spermatocyte (2n)
F - spermatid (n)
G - spermatozoa
H - BM

145. This structure conveys endocrine secretions of the testis into the systemic circulation.

146. This structure secretes an androgenic hormone required for spermatogenesis.

147. This structure releases androgen binding protein which is required for spermatogenesis.

148. This structure is a diploid proliferative cell.

149. This structure contains paired bivalents and it is the site of formation of chiasmata and crossing over.

150. This structure has just completed the first meiotic division.

151. This cell is haploid and is in the early stages of spermiogenesis.

152. This cell is haploid and is in the late stages of spermiogenesis.

153. This cell is the first generation descendant of the primordial germ cell.

154. This cell is the only descendant of the coelomic epithelium in this photomicrograph.

ANSWERS AND TUTORIAL ON ITEMS 145-154

The answers are: **145-A; 146-B; 147-H; 148-C; 149-D; 150-E; 151-F; 152-G; 153-C; 154-I.**
Figure 2.1 shows a high power photomicrograph of a portion of two **seminiferous tubules** in the human adult male. The testis develops from **primordial germ cells** (precursors of gametogenic cell line), coelomic epithelium over urogenital ridge [precursor of **Sertoli cells** (I)], and urogenital ridge mesenchyme (precursor of the tunica albuginea, interstitial vascular and connective tissue, and Leydig cells).

The interstitial tissue between these seminiferous tubules contains a single endocrine **Leydig cell** (B) which is an important source of androgenic steroids such as **testosterone**. The testosterone is conveyed to the systemic circulation via **capillaries** (A) and also diffuses to become concentrated by the action of **androgen binding protein,** which is synthesized in **Sertoli cells** (I) in the seminiferous epithelium and is essential for maintaining the high local androgen concentrations required to support spermatogenesis.

Spermatogenesis begins in diploid (2N DNA, 2N chromatids in 2N chromosomes) proliferative cells called **spermatogonia** (C) which rest on the **basement membrane** (H) of the seminiferous epithelium. Spermatogonia and all of their descendants are derived from primordial germ cells. The spermatogonia are a stem cell population where one daughter remains as a proliferative spermatogonium and the other differentiates into a **primary spermatocyte** (D). Following a round of DNA synthesis and chromatid duplication without centromere division, the primary spermatocyte (4N DNA, 4N chromatids in 2N chromosomes) becomes a tetraploid cell with homologous chromosomes pairing to allow **genetic exchange** between sister chromatids during chiasmata formation. After crossing over, the first meiotic division occurs, producing **secondary spermatocytes** (E) with a haploid number of double chromosomes (2N DNA, 2N chromatids in 1N chromosomes). In the second meiotic division, centromeres divide without either DNA synthesis or chromatid duplication. Once the second meiotic division occurs, **spermatids** (F) are produced which contain 1N DNA, 1N chromatids in 1 N chromosomes. A complex cytomorphogenetic process of **spermiogenesis** then converts the spermatids into **spermatozoa** (G).

Items 155-160

A 15-year-old adolescent presents with a chief complaint of amenorrhea. She is 5'9" tall and weighs 130 lbs. Her temperature is 98.7° F., pulse is 64 beats/min. and blood pressure is 120/60. Physical examination reveals a normal female body habitus except for scant axillary and pubic hair. Pelvic examination reveals a shallow vagina with no cervix. A mobile mass can be palpated in the left labium majorum. Ultrasonographic examination reveals a complete lack of uterus and adnexal structures.

155. The **MOST** appropriate subsequent test to perform for your differential diagnosis is

    (A) laparoscopy
    (B) MRI of pelvis
    (C) karyotype analysis
    (D) glucose tolerance test
    (E) cardiac stress test

156. Which of the following chromosomal complements would you be **MOST** likely to find with this patient after karyotype analysis?

    (A) 45, X
    (B) 47, XX, +21
    (C) 47, XXY
    (D) 46, XY
    (E) 69, XXY

157. The **MOST** appropriate diagnosis is

   (A)   Turner's syndrome
   (B)   Down's syndrome
   (C)   Klinefelter's syndrome
   (D)   androgen insensitivity syndrome
   (E)   triploidy

158. The **MOST** appropriate follow-up procedure indicated is

   (A)   treatment with androgens
   (B)   treatment with estrogens
   (C)   ovariectomy
   (D)   tubal ligation
   (E)   orchiectomy

159. This patient would lack paramesonephric duct derivatives because

   (A)   testes produce müllerian inhibiting substance
   (B)   their differentiation is testosterone dependent
   (C)   the patient is genetically female
   (D)   the patient is genetically male
   (E)   no testis determining factor is produced

160. All of the following statements concerning this patient are true **EXCEPT**:

   (A)   SRY gene present
   (B)   sterility
   (C)   male gender identity
   (D)   degenerate testis present
   (E)   increased risk of seminoma

ANSWERS AND TUTORIAL ON ITEMS 155-160

The answers are: **155-C; 156-D; 157-D; 158-E; 159-A; 160-C**. The most appropriate next test would be a **karyotype analysis** followed by measurements of serum steroids. You would discover that the patient had a 46, XY normal male karyotype and normal testosterone levels. Further tests would reveal a deficiency in testosterone receptor. This patient has **androgen insensitivity** (testicular feminization) **syndrome**. There is an increased risk of seminoma in undescended testes and orchiectomy would be appropriate for the left testicle in the left labium majorum and the right testicle in the inguinal canal or body cavity. While genetically male, this patient would have a female gender identity but would be sterile because of a lack of ovaries and hyalinization of seminiferous epithelium in undescended testes. Because of the presence of a Y chromosome, the **SRY gene** would be present. Paramesonephric duct derivatives (uterine tubes, uterus and upper portion of vagina) would be absent due to müllerian inhibiting substance produced by the undescended and testes.

A 28-year-old woman of Irish ethnic background in the 30th week of her first pregnancy reports a lack of fetal movements. Maternal serum α-fetoprotein levels are significantly elevated. Ultrasonography (**Figure 2.2**) reveals the following (FC = fetal cranium; FCS = fetal cervical spine):

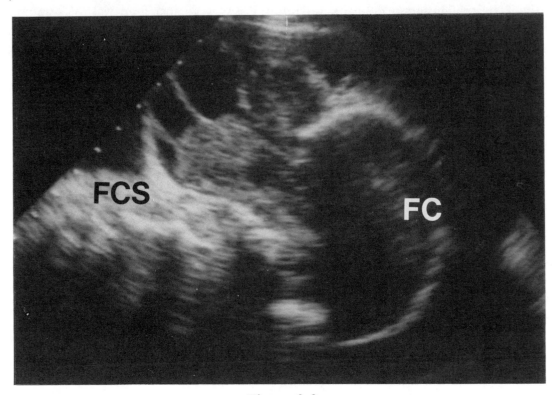

Figure 2.2

161. The **MOST** likely diagnosis of this anomaly is

    (A)   anencephaly
    (B)   spina bifida
    (C)   respiratory distress syndrome
    (D)   spina bifida occulta
    (E)   encephalocele

162. All of the following statements are true concerning this anomaly **EXCEPT**:

   (A)   caused by point mutation
   (B)   likelihood of recurrence of similar congenital anomaly in subsequent pregnancies elevated
   (C)   if carried to term, child has significant risk of paralysis
   (D)   it is a variety of neural tube defect
   (E)   fetus will live after birth

163. The **MOST** appropriate subsequent test for confirmation of diagnosis is

   (A)   assay for amniotic fluid lecithin/sphingomyelin ratio
   (B)   assay for amniotic fluid prostaglandin
   (C)   assay for amniotic fluid α-fetoprotein
   (D)   karyotype analysis of fetal cells
   (E)   karyotype analysis of maternal cells

164. The **MOST** likely developmental process causing this congenital anomaly is

   (A)   failure of neural tube closure
   (B)   failure of lung differentiation
   (C)   duodenal atresia
   (D)   breakage of chromosomes
   (E)   nondisjunction during meiosis

165. The abnormal process causing failure of formation of the skull **MOST** likely is

   (A)   abnormal bone induction
   (B)   excessive production of cerebrospinal fluid
   (C)   inadequate fetal growth
   (D)   formation of amniotic bands
   (E)   abnormal placental transport of calcium

ANSWERS AND TUTORIAL ON ITEMS 161-165

The answers are: **161-E; 162-A; 163-C; 164-A; 165-A**. The ultrasonogram in **Figure 2.2** shows an example of an **encephalocele**. This is a type of **neural tube defect**. Neural tube defects show a complex multifactorial etiology with both genetic and environmental factors contributing to an increased incidence. In this case, the base of the occipital bone is poorly formed. During early development, the neural tube induces formation of the bony structures protecting the central nervous system e.g., the neural arches and the vault of the skull. In many types of neural tube defects, there is both abnormal formation of nervous tissue leading to neurological deficits and abnormal formation of the overlying bony structures normally protecting the nervous system. In encephalocele, meninges protrude into the space created by abnormal formation of the base of the occipital bone. Fetal blood and cerebrospinal fluid contains α-**fetoprotein**. In many neural tube defects, this α-fetoprotein leaks into the amniotic fluid (where it can be measured as an indication of neural tube defects) and may cross into the maternal circulation and subsequently be detected by an assay of maternal serum α-fetoprotein.

Examine the karyotype in **Figure 2.3** below and then answer the items.

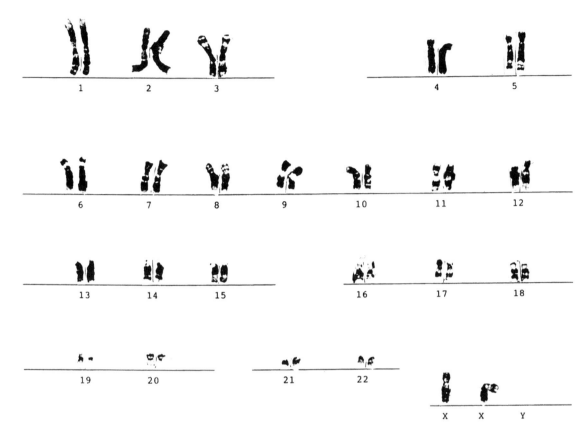

Figure 2.3

166. Which prenatal diagnostic technique is **MOST** commonly used in karyotype analysis?

    (A) ultrasound
    (B) amniocentesis
    (C) fetal heart monitoring
    (D) measurement of maternal serum α-fetoprotein
    (E) urinalysis

167. Which drug is **MOST** commonly used in karyotype analysis?

    (A) steroids
    (B) ß-blockers
    (C) colchicine
    (D) ACTH
    (E) prolactin

168. Which shorthand notation is **MOST** appropriate for describing the karyotype?

   (A)   46, XX
   (B)   47, XXY
   (C)   46, XY
   (D)   45, X
   (E)   45, Y

169. Which statement **BEST** characterizes this karyotype?

   (A)   aneuploidy with numerical anomalies in sex chromosomes
   (B)   aneuploidy with numerical anomalies in autosomes
   (C)   euploidy
   (D)   monosomy
   (E)   trisomy

170. Which of the following disorders would be associated with this karyotype?

   (A)   androgen insensitivity syndrome
   (B)   Klinefelter's syndrome
   (C)   sickle cell anemia
   (D)   Turner's syndrome
   (E)   Down's syndrome

ANSWERS AND TUTORIAL ON ITEMS 166-170

The answers are: **166-B; 167-C; 168-A; 169-C; 170-C. Figure 2.3** is an example of a **normal female karyotype**. Fetal tissue samples must be gathered for karyotype analysis. In prenatal diagnosis, fetal cells can be gathered by amniocentesis or chorionic villus sampling. Following collection of fetal cells, they can be grown in tissue culture. Treatment of cultures of cells with the drug **colchicine** results in the arrest of cell division at metaphase. Chromosomes on the metaphase plate can then be spread, stained, photographed and mounted in a karyotype. This karyotype is a normal female karyotype described by the shorthand notation 46, XX. This is a **euploid** karyotype. Aneuploid karyotypes have numerical anomalies so that there are more or less than 46 chromosomes. Trisomy and monosomy are examples of aneuploid karyotypes. **Klinefelter's syndrome** (47, XXY) is an example of sex chromosome aneuploidy. **Trisomy 21** (Down's syndrome), 47, XX, +21 in a female is an example of an autosomal aneuploidy. **Androgen insensitivity** (testicular feminization) **syndrome** is due to a lack of the testosterone receptor and would be associated with a normal male karyotype (46, XY). **Turner's syndrome** is due to a lack of a second X chromosome (45, X). **Sickle cell anemia** is due to a point mutation in the hemoglobin gene and would be associated with either a normal male or normal female karyotype.

Items 171-175

Examine the karyotype in **Figure 2.4** below and then answer the items.

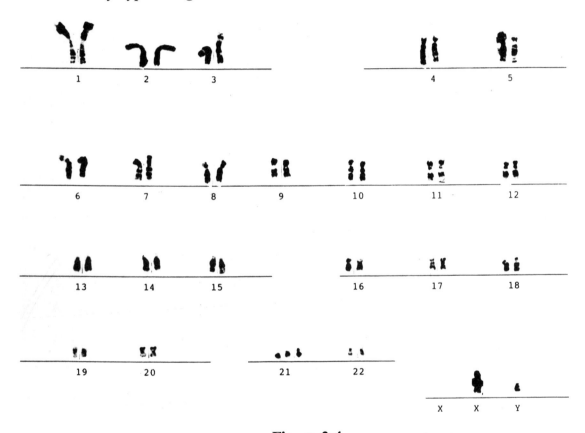

Figure 2.4

171. The developmental process whose disruption produces this karyotype is

    (A)   mitosis
    (B)   synapsis
    (C)   differentiation of primordial germ cells
    (D)   meiotic disjunction
    (E)   migration of primordial germ cells

172. The **BEST** shorthand notation describing this karyotype is

    (A)   46, XY
    (B)   47, XX, +18
    (C)   47, XY, +21
    (D)   47, XXY
    (E)   45, X

173. The **MOST** appropriate diagnosis of a child with this karyotype is

    (A)   Down's syndrome
    (B)   cri-du-chat syndrome
    (C)   Marfan's syndrome
    (D)   Klinefelter's syndrome
    (E)   Turner's syndrome

174. All of the following symptoms and characteristics are associated with this syndrome **EXCEPT**:

    (A)   shortened life expectancy
    (B)   cardiovascular anomalies
    (C)   short stature
    (D)   normal mental function
    (E)   oblique palpebral fissures

175. The **MOST** predictive maternal characteristic for occurrence of this congenital birth defect is

    (A)   alcoholism
    (B)   diabetes mellitus
    (C)   obesity
    (D)   hypertension
    (E)   age greater then 40 years

ANSWERS AND TUTORIAL ON ITEMS 171-175

The answers are: **171-D; 172-C; 173-A; 174-D; 175-E. Figure 2.4** is the karyotype of a male child with **primary nondisjunctional trisomy 21** (Down's syndrome) (47, XY, +21). During synapsis of the first meiotic metaphase, homologous chromosomes pair. If this pairing leads to failure of separation of chromosomes, gametes are produced with either an extra copy of some particular chromosome or the lack of that copy of the chromosome. A human female is born with all of her oocytes arrested in the first meiotic metaphase. Meiosis I is not completed in the human female until just before ovulation. Consequently, synapsis can last for many years. **Increasing maternal age** leads to higher incidence of nondisjunctional chromosomal anomalies including Down's syndrome. When nondisjunction occurs during oogenesis, the ova contain either two copies of chromosome 21 or no copies of chromosome 21, instead of the normal single copy of chromosome 21. When an ovum containing two copies of chromosome 21 is fertilized by a haploid sperm, three copies (2 maternal and one paternal) are found in the zygote and subsequent developmental stages resulting in Down's syndrome. The common symptoms of Down's syndrome are short stature, straight hair, protruding tongue, oblique palpebral fissures and cardiovascular anomalies, e.g., ventricular septal defects. Children with Down's syndrome have a shortened life expectancy and reduced mental function with an IQ around 60.

The common symptoms peculiar to **trisomy 18** (Edwards' syndrome) are microcephaly, prominent occiput, low-set pointed ears, micrognathia, overlapping fingers and rounded feet with a large calcaneus. Cardiovascular and renal defects are also commonly found in Edwards' syndrome but are found in other conditions as well, e.g., cardiovascular defects are also common in Down's syndrome. Children with trisomy 18 usually die soon after birth.

The common symptoms peculiar to **trisomy 13** (Patau's syndrome) are holoprosencephaly, microphthalmia, anophthalmia, cleft lip, cleft palate and polydactyly. Congenital heart defects are found in Patau's syndrome but are found in other conditions as well, e.g., in Down's and Edwards' syndrome. Children with trisomy 13 usually die soon after birth.

Items 176-179

A fetus is delivered at 32 weeks since the last menstrual period. At birth, the fetus weighs 1500 gm but otherwise appears normal. Soon after birth, however, the fetus becomes cyanotic and breathes with a grunting noise. Chest X-rays reveal dense lungs with significant atelectasis. Choose the **BEST** response.

176. The **MOST** likely diagnosis associated with these symptoms is

    (A)   congenital diaphragmatic hernia
    (B)   coarctation of the aorta
    (C)   tetralogy of Fallot
    (D)   renal agenesis
    (E)   respiratory distress syndrome

177. The **MOST** significant predictive prenatal test for this disease would be

    (A)   ultrasonography
    (B)   X-rays
    (C)   measurement of amniotic fluid lecithin/sphingomyelin ratio
    (D)   karyotype analysis
    (E)   measurement of maternal serum α-fetoprotein

178. The cell type **MOST** directly involved in etiology of this condition is

    (A)   type I pneumocyte
    (B)   type II pneumocyte
    (C)   macrophage
    (D)   erythrocyte
    (E)   capillary endothelium

179. In threatened premature delivery, the **MOST** useful drug class for treatment of the mother to accelerate fetal lung maturation is

    (A)   antibiotic
    (B)   antimetabolite
    (C)   neuroleptic
    (D)   steroid
    (E)   diuretic

ANSWERS AND TUTORIAL ON ITEMS 176-179

The answers are: **176-E; 177-C; 178-A; 179-D**. The leading cause of death among premature infants is **respiratory distress syndrome**. A fetus 30 weeks from the last menstrual period is 28 weeks gestational age. At 28 weeks gestational age, **type II pneumocytes** have only just begun to differentiate and secrete surfactant. The most abundant phospholipid in surfactant is **lecithin**. The sphingomyelin levels in amniotic fluid are relatively constant throughout gestation but the lecithin levels begin to rise slowly at 28 weeks. Once many type II cells differentiate, they secrete substantial quantities of surfactant which enters the amniotic fluid during to fetal respiratory movements. Due to increasing surfactant secretion, the lecithin/sphingomyelin ratio increases. Type II cell differentiation is a steroid-dependent process. Treatment of women with certain steroid drugs will stimulate precocious differentiation of type II cells and thus reduce the risk of respiratory distress syndrome in premature infants.

You are asked to evaluate a newborn infant who has had a low Apgar score and still has inadequate color on weak crying 2 hours after birth, despite suctioning and Ambulatory Mechanical Breathing Unit (AMBU) ventilation. AP (**Figure 2.5A**) and lateral (**Figure 2.5B**) chest X-rays are obtained and brought to you as you listen for breath sounds in the chest.

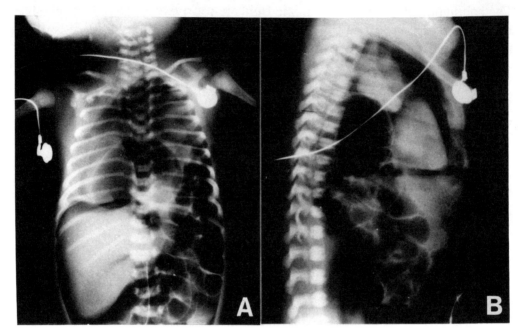

Figure 2.5

180. The **MOST** likely diagnosis is

    (A)   pulmonary sequestration
    (B)   meconium aspiration
    (C)   tracheoesophageal fistula
    (D)   diaphragmatic hernia
    (E)   tension pneumothorax

181. The next **MOST** likely complication to develop if this problem is untreated is

    (A)   hemorrhage
    (B)   perforation
    (C)   hypoxic arrest
    (D)   short gut syndrome
    (E)   organizing pneumonia

182. This congenital anomaly is due to failure of proper morphogenesis of which of the following structures?

(A) pericardioperitoneal fold
(B) pleuroperitoneal fold
(C) pleuropericardial fold
(D) dorsal mesoesophagus
(E) septum transversum

183. Survival of infants born with a diaphragmatic hernia is **MOST** dependent on

(A) time to recognition of disease
(B) degree of pulmonary hypoplasia
(C) adequacy of antibiotic coverage
(D) capacitance of abdominal cavity
(E) oxygen toxicity

ANSWERS AND TUTORIAL ON ITEMS 180-183

The answers are: **180-D; 181-C; 182-B; 183-B**. The chest X-ray films in **Figure 2.5** show a newborn with **congenital diaphragmatic hernia** (of Bochdalek). Normally, the diaphragm forms by the fusion of 4 rudiments:

1) septum transversum
2) dorsal mesoesophagus
3) **pleuroperitoneal folds**
4) muscular ingrowth from the body wall

When the pleuroperitoneal folds fail to form properly, more often on the left than right side, a large opening called the **foramen of Bochdalek** develops in the posterolateral region of the diaphragm.

In this patient, substantial small bowel loops are present in the thoracic cavity through the incomplete separation of the pleural and peritoneal cavities by the congenital diaphragmatic defect. The presence of the bowel in the chest hinders formation of the lungs leading to **pulmonary hypoplasia** which decreases the alveolar surface area for gas exchange. In some instances the developing heart is shifted to the right and may also exhibit congenital defects. Even with suctioning, positive pressure ventilation, and intubation, the newborn's skin does not become pink. Because the persistent hypoxia, hypoxic arrest is a likely outcome. Since the defect is large, incarceration of abdominal viscera within the chest is unlikely. Although the viscera that have become resident in the chest have "lost domain" and the peritoneal capacitance may be decreased, the rate-limiting feature of diaphragmatic hernia is the concomitant failure of pulmonary development. The **degree of pulmonary hypoplasia** is often the feature that determines survival in such infants in whom abdominal viscera are returned to the abdomen and the diaphragmatic hernia is repaired surgically. The adequacy of the lungs to maintain oxygenated blood in the newborn is mainly a function of the degree of pulmonary hypoplasia. Sometimes this condition may require extrapulmonary oxygenation such as with extracorporeal membrane oxygenator use.

Items 184-195

Examine the labeled scanning electron micrograph of a human embryo in **Figure 2.6** below and then match each of the statements below with the **MOST** appropriate lettered structure in the micrograph. Lettered structures may be used once, more than once, or not at all.

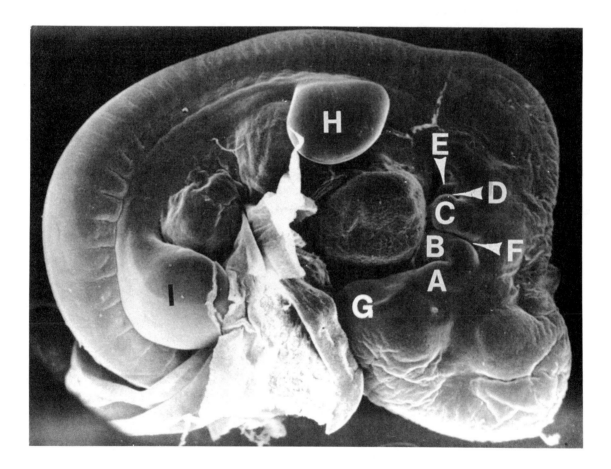

Figure 2.6

184. Developmental anomalies in this structure cause the mandibular hypoplasia seen in mandibulofacial dysostosis (Treacher Collins syndrome).

185. The mesenchyme in this structure forms the maxilla.

186. The aortic arch in this pharyngeal arch forms the hyoid and stapedial arteries in the adult.

187. This structure forms the external auditory canal in the adult.

188. Meckel's cartilage forms in the mesenchyme of this structure.

189. The aortic arch in this structure gives rise to part of the internal carotid artery.

190. The masseter and temporalis muscles differentiate in the mesoderm of this structure.

191. Micrognathia results from hypoplasia of this structure.

192. The styloid process, stylohyoid ligament and lesser horn of the hyoid bone are remnants of the cartilage in this structure.

193. The central portion of the forehead and the frontal bone is formed in this structure.

Choose the **BEST** response.

194. All of the following statements about pharyngeal arches are true **EXCEPT**:

    (A) The arches contain mesenchyme derived from neural crest cells.
    (B) Skeletal structures in the arches are derived from neural crest cells.
    (C) Arch-derived skeletal muscles arise *in situ* from somitomeres.
    (D) The amount of adult tissue derived from each arch is equal.
    (E) The vascular endothelium is derived from the resident mesoderm.

195. The laryngeal cartilages form in which pharyngeal structure?

    (A) second pouch
    (B) second arch mesenchyme
    (C) third pouch
    (D) third arch mesenchyme
    (E) fourth arch mesenchyme

The answers are: **184-B; 185-A; 186-C; 187-F; 188-B; 189-D; 190-B; 191-B; 192-C; 193-G; 194-D; 195-E**. **Figure 2.6** is a scanning electron micrograph of a human embryo of approximately 5 weeks after fertilization. The first pharyngeal arch is divided into a **maxillary prominence** (A) and a **mandibular prominence** (B). The **first pharyngeal groove** (F) is clearly visible between the first and **second** (C) **pharyngeal arches**.

The mesenchyme in the maxillary prominence will form the maxilla. The mesenchyme in the mandibular prominence will form Meckel's cartilage and eventually the mandible. Micrognathia would result from abnormal development of the mandible. **Mandibulofacial dysostosis** (first arch syndrome, Treacher Collins syndrome) is caused by an autosomal dominant mutation with a sex ratio of 1:1. This mutation causes developmental anomalies in derivatives of the first pharyngeal arch. The major clinical findings associated with this anomaly are downward slanting palpebral fissures, malar hypoplasia, microtia and conductive hearing loss due to abnormalities in the auditory ossicles and external auditory meatus. This hearing loss is often misdiagnosed as mental retardation which is not a characteristic of people with mandibulofacial dysostosis. The muscles of mastication, e.g., masseter and temporalis muscles, are formed in first arch mesenchyme and are innervated by the mandibular division of the Vth (trigeminal) cranial nerve. The aortic arches of the first and second pharyngeal arches undergo extensive degenerative changes during development but persist in the adult as the maxillary artery (first arch) and hyoid and stapedial artery (second arch). The first pharyngeal groove gives rise to the external auditory canal while the **first pharyngeal pouch** forms the auditory tube.

The **second pharyngeal arch** (C) forms the muscles of facial expression, e.g., the orbicularis oris and orbicularis oculi. The muscles of facial expression are innervated by the VIIth cranial nerve (facial nerve). The **second aortic arch** forms the hyoid and stapedial arteries. The **second** (D) and more caudal **pharyngeal grooves** disappear due to caudal overgrowth by the second pharyngeal arch. The **second pharyngeal pouch** forms the fossa of the palatine tonsils.

The **third pharyngeal arch** (E) is also visible. Both the third and fourth pouches contribute to the parathyroid glands while the thymus is derived from the third pharyngeal arch only. The **third aortic arch** forms a portion of the internal carotid artery. The rest of the internal carotid artery is derived from the dorsal aorta. The fourth pharyngeal arch has disappeared in this embryo. The mesoderm of the fourth pharyngeal arch forms the laryngeal cartilages.

Tissues traditionally thought of as solely mesodermal in origin are also derived from neural crest cells in the head and neck. Head mesenchyme and pharyngeal arch cartilages are derived from neural crest. Skeletal muscles and vascular endothelium apparently arise from somite-like (not completely segmented) masses of paraxial mesoderm called **somitomeres**.

The **frontal prominence** (G) will become the forehead. The frontal bone forms in the mesenchyme of the frontal prominence by intramembranous ossification, i.e., without a preformed cartilaginous model. The **forelimb bud** (H) and **hindlimb bud** (I) are both visible.

For the convenience of the reader, the basic adult derivatives of the different components of the pharyngeal apparatus are summarized in **Table 2.1** below:

TABLE 2.1

SUMMARY OF ADULT STRUCTURES DERIVED FROM PHARYNGEAL ARCHES

Pharyngeal Arch	Arch Derivatives			Pouch Derivatives	Groove Derivatives	Nerve Supply
	Muscles	Skeletal Structures	Ligaments			
First (mandibular)	Mastication muscles Mylohyoid Anterior belly of digastric Tensor tympani Tensor veli palatini	(Meckel's cartilage) Malleus Incus ventral end of mandible	Anterior ligament of malleus Sphenomandibular ligament	Tubotympanic recess (tympanic membrane, tympanic cavity, mastoid antrum, auditory tube)	External auditory canal	V (trigeminal)
Second (hyoid)	Facial expression muscles Stapedius Stylohyoid Posterior belly of digastric	(Reichert's cartilage) Stapes Styloid process Hyoid bone (lesser horn and upper body)	Stylohyoid ligament	Tonsilar fossa	None	VII (facial)
Third	Stylopharyngeus	Hyoid bone (greater horn and lower body)	None	Inferior parathyroid Thymus	None	IX (glossopharyngeal)
Fourth and sixth combined	Cricothyroid Levator veli palatini Constrictors of pharynx Intrinsic muscles of larynx	Laryngeal cartilages (cricoid, thyroid, arytenoid, corniculate, cuneiform)	None	Superior parathyroids Ultimobra		

Examine the child shown in **Figure 2.7**. Then choose the **BEST** response to the items below.

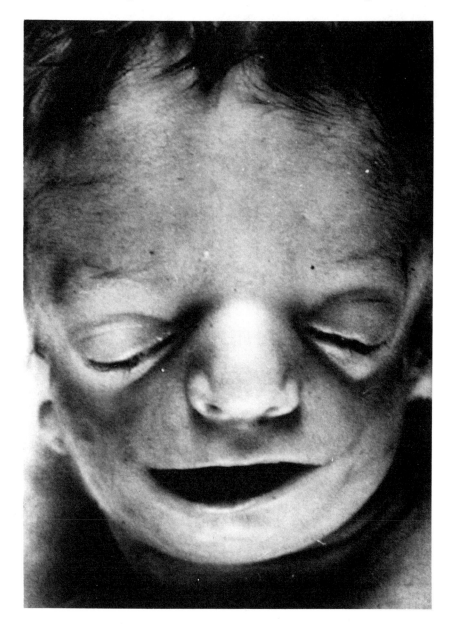

Figure 2.7

196. This child is **MOST** likely afflicted with which of the following conditions?

   (A)   fetal alcohol syndrome
   (B)   trisomy 21
   (C)   DiGeorge syndrome
   (D)   Treacher Collins syndrome
   (E)   trisomy 18

197. All of the following statements concerning this condition are correct **EXCEPT**:

   (A)   probably caused by one or more autosomal dominant genes
   (B)   often associated with deformities of the ears
   (C)   often associated with down slanting palpebral fissures
   (D)   often associated with poorly developed zygomatic bones
   (E)   condition precludes a normal life span

198. Individuals with this condition

   (A)   Exhibit maldevelopment of mainly second pharyngeal arch components.
   (B)   Rarely exhibit irregular tooth eruption even through the mouth is often large.
   (C)   Often exhibit hypoplasia of the hyoid apparatus resulting in swallowing difficulties.
   (D)   Typically exhibit mandibulofacial dysostosis.
   (E)   Probably produced supernumerary neural crest cells during the embryonic period.

ANSWERS AND TUTORIAL ON ITEMS 196-198

The answers are: **196-D; 197-E; 198-D**. Individuals with **mandibulofacial dysostosis** (Treacher Collins syndrome, first arch syndrome) (an example of which is shown in **Figure 2.7**) have a normal life span and normal mental capacity. All of the other choices are correct. This condition is a manifestation of first arch dysgenesis accompanied by maxillary and mandibular hypoplasia and malocclusion from irregular tooth eruption. The syndrome is thought to be caused by insufficient production of neural crest cells.

Items 199-200

A mother and her two year-old son come to your office. The mother complains that the child is not acting normally. After a brief period of active play, her son becomes exhausted, breathes rapidly and squats or lies down. On physical examination, you find that the child's pulse and blood pressure are normal. His oral mucosa, fingernails and toenails are cyanotic. You also detect a significant systolic murmur best heard along the left sternal border at the level of the second intercostal space. A PA (posteroanterior) chest film shows a concavity on the left border of the heart, diminished pulmonary vascularity and a rounded heart apex located slightly higher than normal above the diaphragm.

199.   The **MOST** likely diagnosis of the boy's problem is

     (A)   isolated ventricular septal defect
     (B)   isolated atrial septal defect
     (C)   isolated aortic stenosis
     (D)   transposition of the great vessels
     (E)   tetralogy of Fallot

200.   All of the following are common anatomical features of this condition **EXCEPT**:

     (A)   pulmonary stenosis
     (B)   left ventricular hypertrophy
     (C)   overriding aorta
     (D)   ventricular septal defect
     (E)   patent ductus arteriosus

ANSWERS AND TUTORIAL ON ITEMS 199-200

The answers are: **199-E; 200-B**. This child has the **tetralogy of Fallot**. The mild cyanosis and dyspnea are caused by the poor vascular perfusion of the lungs due to the **pulmonary artery stenosis** and **ventricular septal defect** with large right to left shunt. Abnormally high pressure in the right ventricle due to the **overriding aorta** causes **right ventricular hypertrophy** and is largely responsible for the radiological findings. The **systolic murmur** is due to turbulence of blood flow through the right ventricular outflow tract.

The primitive heart, prior to ventricular septation, has a single large ventricle which leads into a large ventricular outflow tract called the **conus cordis**. The conus cordis leads into the **truncus arteriosus** which in turn supplies blood to the aortic sac and **aortic arches**. The tetralogy of Fallot is the most frequently seen abnormality caused by unequal division of the conus cordis and truncus arteriosus. This defect is caused by an anterior displacement of the **truncoconal septum**, a flap of tissue that forms in the conus cordis and truncus arteriosus to divided the ventricular outflow tracts. Prior to birth, the **ductus arteriosus**, a derivative of the left distal 6th aortic arch, provides a shunt between the pulmonary and the systemic circulation. Soon after birth, the ductus arteriosus closes and degenerates, leaving behind a **ligamentum arteriosum**. In many cases of tetralogy of Fallot, there is also a persistent ductus arteriosus.

Items 201-207

Match each of the descriptions relating to heart development in the items below with the **MOST** appropriate lettered structure in **Figure 2.8** below. Each answer may be used once, more than once, or not at all.

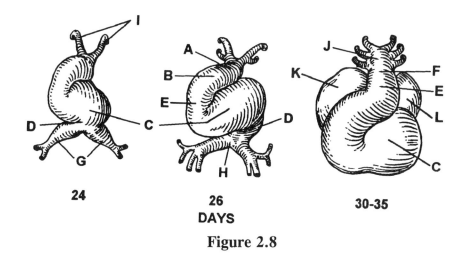

Figure 2.8

201. Gives rise to the ascending aorta and pulmonary trunk.

202. Gives rise to most of the trabeculated part of the right ventricle.

203. Gives rise to the smooth-walled part of the right atrium.

87

204.   Region known as the conus cordis.

205.   Represents first aortic arch.

206.   Region known as the primitive atrium.

207.   Region which receives the two vitelline veins.

ANSWERS AND TUTORIAL ON ITEMS 201-207

The answers are: **201-F; 202-B; 203-H; 204-E; 205-I; 206-D; 207-H**. **Figure 2.8** illustrates the early development of the human heart. The **sinus venosus** (H) is a symmetric expansion of the caudal end of the primitive heart tube consisting of a median region and a **left and right sinus horn** (G). The **vitelline**, umbilical, and common cardinal veins open into the sinus venosus. The sinus venosus gives rise to the smooth-walled part of the **definitive right atrium**. The part of the right atrial wall with pectinate muscles (anterior to the crista terminalis) and the right and left auricles are derived from the primitive atrium. The **primitive ventricle** (C) gives rise to most of the **definitive left ventricle** and is separated from the primitive atrium by an atrioventricular sulcus. The bulbus cordis differentiates into several structures and is separated from the ventricle by the bulboventricular sulcus. The most caudal region of the **bulbus cordis** (B) forms the trabeculated part of the **right ventricle**. The rest of the bulbus cordis, called the **conus cordis** (E), contributes to the formation of two definitive outflow tracts of the ventricles called the infundibulum of the right ventricle and the aortic vestibule of the left ventricle. The **truncus arteriosus** (F) forms the **ascending aorta** and the **pulmonary trunk**. The **aortic sac** (J) is cranial to the heart tube and connects directly to the **first aortic arches** (I). The other aortic arches will arise from the aortic sac.

Match the lettered structures in **Figure 2.9** below with the **CORRECT** statement regarding developmental fate in the items below. Answers may be used once, more than once, or not at all.

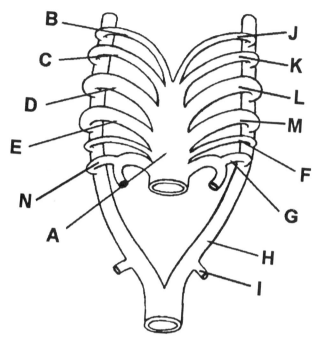

Figure 2.9

208.   Gives rise to the ductus arteriosus.

209.   Gives rise to right common carotid and right proximal internal carotid artery.

210.   Along with the right 7th intersegmental and a portion of the right dorsal aorta, this arch will form the right subclavian artery.

211.   In humans, this aortic arch never develops or exists only briefly and does not contribute to any definitive artery.

212.   Gives rise to the proximal part of the arch of the aorta.

213.   Gives rise to the right maxillary artery.

214.   The right recurrent laryngeal nerve loops around the derivative of this aortic arch.

ANSWERS AND TUTORIAL ON ITEMS 208-214

The answers are: **208-G; 209-D; 210-E; 211-F; 212-A; 213-B; 214-E**. During development four well-defined pairs of pharyngeal arches appear externally in humans. Each arch contains an artery called an **aortic arch (Figure 2.9)**. Each arch arises from the **aortic sac** and courses dorsally to the left or right dorsal aorta. The four pairs of arches, numbered 1 through 4, persist to give rise to definitive structures. Based primarily on the ontogeny of lower forms, fifth and sixth pharyngeal arches have been described but in the human embryo they are vestigial

The **truncus arteriosus** and **aortic sac** (A) develop into the **ascending aorta.** The aortic sac also forms the proximal portion of the **arch of the aorta.** The right and left dorsal aortae fuse during the 4th week to form a midline **dorsal aorta,** which later becomes the **descending aorta.** Remnants of aortic arches 1 and 2 give rise to minor vascular elements in the head. The **1st arch** (B, J) forms the terminal segment of the **maxillary artery.** The **2nd arch** (C, K) forms the stapedial artery. **Arches 3 and 4** give rise to important vessels of the head, neck and upper thorax. The **3rd arch** (D, L) will supply blood to the head. Earlier, the head was supplied by the cranial portions of the paired dorsal aortae, but the segments of the dorsal aortae between the 3rd and 4th arches degenerate. The 3rd arch becomes the **common carotid artery** and the **beginning portion of the internal carotid artery**. The distal portion of the internal carotid artery develops from the original dorsal aorta. The **external carotid artery** arises *de novo* from the internal carotid artery.

The **4th arch** (E, M) becomes part of the **arch of the aorta** on the left side and the **subclavian artery** on the right side. Initially, the upper limb receives the seventh cervical intersegmental artery (I), a branch of the dorsal aorta. On the left side, the **left 4th aortic arch** becomes the middle portion of the arch of the aorta. The **left 7th intersegmental artery** becomes the **left subclavian artery.** On the right side, the **right 4th arch** becomes the root of the **right subclavian artery**. The portion of the right dorsal aorta between the right 7th intersegmental artery and the descending aorta degenerates. The **brachiocephalic artery** develops from a portion of the aortic sac.

The precursor of the distal part of the **pulmonary trunk** and the **ductus arteriosus** is often described as a **left sixth arch** (G). The right and left pulmonary arteries originate as branches from the 4th arch but later shift their origin to the pulmonary trunk.

The asymmetrical development of the 4th and 6th arches explains the differing courses of the right and left recurrent laryngeal nerves. On the right side the 5th and 6th arches never form, so the **right recurrent laryngeal nerve** comes to loop around the right subclavian artery, the derivative of the **right 4th arch.** On the left, the 6th arch becomes the ductus arteriosus and thus the **left recurrent laryngeal** loops around this **6th arch** derivative.

90

During a routine obstetrical examination, you find that your patient has an abnormally small abdominal girth for her 30 week pregnancy. Ultrasonographic examination reveals a normal fetus, a posterior fundal placenta and oligohydramnios.

215.   The decreased volume of amniotic fluid (oligohydramnios) could be caused by which of the following?

   (A)   renal agenesis
   (B)   bladder exstrophy
   (C)   anencephaly
   (D)   tracheoesophageal fistula
   (E)   duodenal torsion

216.   The **MOST** likely fundamental developmental defect leading to this clinical case is failed

   (A)   ureteric bud induction
   (B)   cloacal membrane septation
   (C)   neural tube closure
   (D)   secondary canalization
   (E)   mid-gut loop rotation

ANSWERS AND TUTORIAL ON ITEMS 215-216

The answers are: **215-A; 216-A**. Complete **renal agenesis** most likely results from a failure of development of the metanephric (definitive) kidney. The fundamental process leading to formation of the **metanephros** is a reciprocal inductive interaction between the **ureteric bud** (a branch of the mesonephric duct) and the **metanephric blastema** (the caudal portion of the urogenital ridge). The ureteric bud grows into the metanephric blastema and is induced to branch many times leading to the formation of the ureters, major calyces, minor calyces and collecting ducts of the definitive kidney. The ureteric bud induces the formation of nephrons in the metanephric blastema. Derivatives of the metanephric blastema include the renal glomerulus and other blood vessels, connective tissue, Bowman's capsule, proximal convoluted tubule, loop of Henle and distal convoluted tubule.
       The fetus normally produces a small amount of hypotonic urine and urinates it into the amniotic fluid. Subsequently, the fetus swallows the amniotic fluid. Renal agenesis results in no urine formation and therefore a reduction in volume of amniotic fluid (**oligohydramnios**). Anencephalic fetuses have no swallowing function but do produce urine, leading to the excessive

volume of amniotic fluid (**polyhydramnios**). Urine production is normal in bladder exstrophy which does not become apparent as a clinical problem until after birth. Blockage of the gastrointestinal tract would also lead to polyhydramnios.

Items 217-218

A 42-year-old pregnant woman has chorionic villus sampling performed for cytogenetic analysis of her fetus. The scanning electron micrograph in **Figure 2.10** is prepared from this sample. Examine this micrograph and then answer the items concerning the developing placenta.

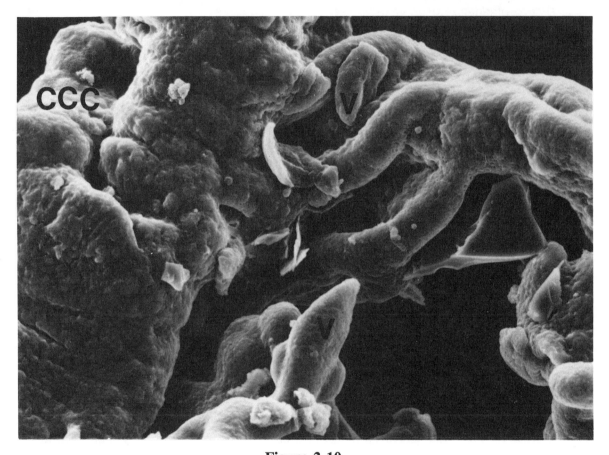

Figure 2.10

217. The cytotrophoblastic cell columns (CCC) have all of the following morphological characteristics **EXCEPT**:

(A) fetal blood vessels
(B) maternal blood vessels
(C) connective tissue
(D) cytotrophoblast
(E) syncytiotrophoblast

218. The villi (V) have all of the following morphological characteristics **EXCEPT**:

(A)   a continuous layer of cytotrophoblastic cells
(B)   a continuous syncytiotrophoblast
(C)   a connective tissue core
(D)   decidual cells
(E)   they are bathed in maternal blood

ANSWERS AND TUTORIAL ON ITEMS 217-218

The answers are: **217-B; 218-D**. **Figure 2.10** is a scanning electron micrograph of a sample of **chorionic villi**. Chorionic villus sampling is gradually replacing amniocentesis as a technique for gathering fetal tissue for cytogenetic analysis. This technique has several advantages. First, it can be performed earlier than amniocentesis and thus can give diagnosis of cytogenetic or biochemical abnormalities at an earlier stage in pregnancy. It also yields samples of rapidly growing fetal tissue which can be grown into substantial numbers of cells for karyotype or biochemical analysis more easily and more rapidly than fetal tissue samples collected by amniocentesis. **Cytotrophoblastic cell columns** (CCC) connect the chorionic plate and the basal (decidual) plate of the developing placenta. They consist of columns of fetal connective tissue surrounding fetal blood vessels. The cytotrophoblastic cell columns are covered by the layer of cytotrophoblastic cells and a layer of syncytiotrophoblast. They contain no maternal blood vessels. **Chorionic villi** (V) project from the cytotrophoblastic cell columns into the intervillous spaces. Villi are bathed in maternal blood that enters the intervillous spaces through branches of the uterine artery that penetrate the basal (decidual) plate. Villi also contain fetal blood vessels surrounded by fetal connective tissue. The villi are coated by a layer of cytotrophoblast and syncytiotrophoblast. Maternal decidual tissue is found in the placenta but not in the villi proper.

A 37-year-old 148 lb woman is found to be carrying monoamnionic twins. In spite of complete continuous bed rest from 28 weeks after conception, she is found to have ruptured membranes at 34 weeks. Two days after rupture of membranes, maternal temperature is 103° F. and her white blood count is 20,000/mm^3 with a predominance of neutrophils. Your diagnosis is chorioamnionitis.

Choose the **BEST** response.

219.   The chief morphological change in the fetal lymph nodes as a result of this intrauterine infection would be

   (A)   ingression
   (B)   increase in T-cells
   (C)   infiltration by neutrophils
   (D)   appearance of eosinophils
   (E)   appearance of germinal centers

220.   These morphological changes are a reflection of which immunological process?

   (A)   T-cell proliferation
   (B)   activation of memory B-cells
   (C)   delayed hypersensitivity
   (D)   plasma cell phagocytosis
   (E)   B-cell activation and differentiation

221.   Which mechanism is **MOST** important for passive immunization of the fetus against antigenic exposure of the mother prior to birth?

   (A)   placental transport of maternal IgGs
   (B)   synthesis of secretory IgAs
   (C)   placental transport of maternal IgMs
   (D)   colostrum formation
   (E)   placental transport of IgEs

The answers are: **219-E; 220-E; 221-A**. Premature rupture of fetal membranes often leads to **chorioamnionitis** with elevated temperature and elevated white blood cell count. The normal white blood cell count is approximately 5,000/mm³. Under normal circumstances, the fetus develops in a sterile environment and is therefore not exposed to bacterial antigens. Consequently, fetal lymph nodes lack germinal centers. At birth, the fetus is suddenly exposed to an entire new population of bacterial antigens. This potential problem is dealt with in three ways. First, during gestation, the fetus is passively immunized against bacterial antigens by **transplacental transport** of maternal **IgGs**. Higher molecular weight IgM is not transported across the placenta. Second, if the child is breast fed, **colostrum** contains high concentrations of secretory IgAs that bind to enteric bacteria and prevent their adhesion to the gastrointestinal epithelium. Third, once the fetus becomes exposed to bacterial antigens, his or her own lymph nodes (if antigens are lymph-born) and spleen (if the antigens are blood-born) become activated. Germinal centers represent areas where B-lymphocytes, in conjunction with helper T-cells and antigen-presenting macrophages are becoming activated. This activation involves decreasing nuclear condensation and increasing cytoplasm to produce the intracellular machinery for IgG synthesis. Once stimulated, B-cells differentiate into immunoglobulin secreting **plasma cells**. Germinal centers also contain large numbers of macrophages.

Items 222-225

In a second pregnancy, a 25-year-old woman delivers a hydropic fetus with severe edema, jaundice and hepatosplenomegaly. Her blood type is O negative and her husband's blood type is O positive.

Choose the **BEST** response.

222.   The blood type of the fetus is

    (A)   A negative
    (B)   A positive
    (C)   O negative
    (D)   O positive
    (E)   B positive

223. All of the following statements concerning the fetal red blood cells are correct **EXCEPT**:

   (A)   they lack Rh antigen
   (B)   they are destroyed in the fetal spleen
   (C)   they are produced in the fetal liver
   (D)   they are produced in fetal bone marrow
   (E)   they are coated with maternally derived IgG

224. The **MOST** appropriate description of the cause of fetal hepatosplenomegaly is

   (A)   Maternal IgGs cause stimulation of Kupffer cells.
   (B)   Liver and spleen enlarge to facilitate removal of hemoglobin degradation products.
   (C)   These organs are active in destruction and production of fetal red blood cells.
   (D)   Fetal blood volume increased so these organs have more blood in them than usual.
   (E)   Spleen and liver show hypertrophy to substitute for compromised placental function.

225. The **PRIMARY** cause of Rh isoimmunization is

   (A)   leakage of fetal RBCs into maternal blood supply
   (B)   accumulation of fetal IgGs at placenta
   (C)   failure of transplacental transport of maternal IgGs to fetus
   (D)   immunization of mother against paternal spermatozoa
   (E)   abnormal hepatic morphogenesis

ANSWERS AND TUTORIAL ON ITEMS 222-225

The answers are: **222-D; 223-A; 224-C; 225-A. Rh isoimmunization** occurs in fetuses with Rh-mothers and Rh+ fathers. The Rh antigen is controlled by a dominant gene and therefore the fetus of an Rh- mother and Rh+ father would be Rh+. Rh isoimmunization is more severe with each pregnancy because the maternal immune system has a memory for Rh isoimmunization. Normally, the placental trophoblast serves as a barrier between fetal and maternal blood, although microvascular accidents allowing mixture of fetal and maternal blood are inevitable. When fetal RBCs leak into the maternal blood supply, they are recognized as foreign antigens by the maternal immune system. Maternal IgGs are produced against the fetal RBCs and these are transported functionally intact across the placenta into the fetal circulatory system. Here, these IgGs bind to fetal RBCs and cause their destruction in the fetal liver and spleen. The resulting anemia stimulates fetal erythropoiesis in the bone marrow, liver and spleen. Consequently, enlargement of the liver and spleen occurs. Excessive destruction of fetal RBCs results in accumulation of bile pigments and thus **jaundice**.

You are a Public Health Service pediatrician working on a rural health clinic in Mississippi. A 35-year-old woman with hepatomegaly and facial spider angiomas visits your clinic with her 5-year-old son. The mother admits to heavy drinking on a regular basis but denies alcohol consumption during her pregnancy. The child, shown in **Figure 2.11** below, is short for his age and shows significant mid-facial hypoplasia, including ocular ptosis and a flat nasal bridge. The child seems lethargic and there is a significant deficit in his social interactions.

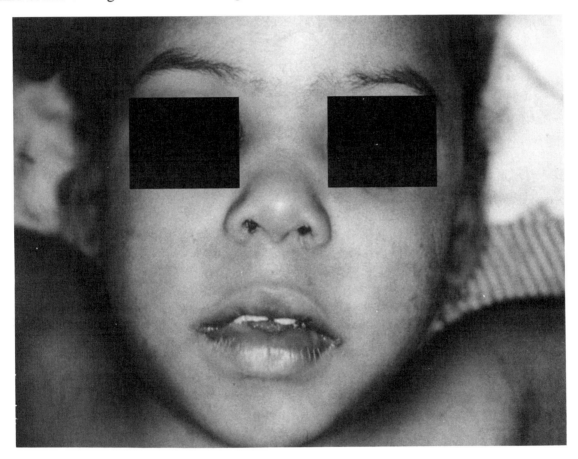

Figure 2.11

226. The **MOST** likely diagnosis of the maternal-child disease is

    (A)   healthy-Down's syndrome
    (B)   healthy-Treacher Collins syndrome
    (C)   alcoholism-fetal alcohol syndrome
    (D)   alcoholism-vitamin B_{12} deficiency
    (E)   alcoholism-pellagra

227. The **MOST** likely defective developmental process that lead to the child's symptoms is

(A)　neural crest cell migration
(B)　bone formation
(C)　ocular induction
(D)　cartilage proliferation
(E)　endochondral ossification

ANSWERS AND TUTORIAL ON ITEMS 226-227

The answers are: **226-C; 227-A.** There is a high probability that the mother is an alcoholic. Her obesity, hepatomegaly and spider angiomas are highly suggestive of alcoholism. Her denial of alcohol consumption during pregnancy is suspect. The child in **Figure 2.11** shows many of the features of **fetal alcohol syndrome** (FAS) including short stature, facial abnormalities and mild mental retardation. Alcohol and acetaldehyde are known teratogens. They cross the placenta rapidly and persist in the fetus long after being cleared from the maternal system. The fetal hepatic detoxification functions for alcohol are poorly developed. Experimental studies in mammalian embryos suggest that one of the primary causative events in FAS teratogenesis is inhibition of cell migration. Neural crest cells migrate into the pharyngeal apparatus where they participate in morphogenesis of facial bones. The mid-facial hypoplasia characteristic of FAS children is most likely due to defects in neural crest cell migration.

A new-born infant fails to defecate for 3 days after birth in spite of normal feeding without excessive vomiting. Rectal examination reveals a normal rectum but a fecal mass retained in the colon. There is an explosive release of feces following cessation of rectal examination. Barium enema and x-rays reveals a narrowed distal segment of the colon and a dilated proximal segment.

228.   The **MOST** likely diagnosis of this condition is

   (A)   sprue
   (B)   colic
   (C)   colonic aganglionosis
   (D)   imperforate anus
   (E)   gastric atresia

229.   The **MOST** likely developmental abnormality leading to this condition is

   (A)   gluten allergy
   (B)   abnormal gastric rotation
   (C)   abnormal neural crest cell migration
   (D)   failure of proctodeal membrane degeneration
   (E)   situs inversus

ANSWERS AND TUTORIAL ON ITEMS 228-229

The answers are: **228-C; 229-C**. This patient is suffering from **Hirschsprung's disease** or colonic aganglionosis. Biopsy of the distal colon would reveal that the parasympathetic ganglia and other neuronal elements of the myenteric plexus are absent from the narrowed portion of the colon. Ganglia are present in the distended portion of the colon. The neurons of the myenteric plexus are derived from the **neural crest** and the congenital anomaly is due to abnormal neural crest cell migration to the colon. Neural crest cells also contribute to dorsal root ganglia; form the adrenal medulla; form Schwann cells, myelinating cells in the peripheral nervous system; form meninges; form melanocytes; and form odontoblasts, the dentin-secreting cells of tooth germs.

Contrast media can be injected into blood vessels to reveal by x-ray the blood flow from one vessel to another. In the hemochorial human placenta, a contrast dye is injected into either the uterine artery or the umbilical vein and 10 seconds later the dye is located by radiography.

230. The vascular space **MOST** intensely labeled immediately after injection of contrast medium into the uterine artery is/are the

(A) umbilical artery
(B) umbilical vein
(C) capillaries in the chorionic villi
(D) intervillous space
(E) uterine vein

231. The vascular space **MOST** intensely labeled immediately after injection of contrast medium into the umbilical vein is the

(A) inferior vena cava
(B) ductus venosus
(C) ductus arteriosus
(D) umbilical artery
(E) superior vena cava

ANSWERS AND TUTORIAL ON ITEMS 230-231

The answers are: **230-D; 231-B**. Maternal oxygenated blood is supplied to the placenta from branches of the **uterine arteries**. These vessels empty into the intervillous space where they carry oxygen to and remove carbon dioxide from capillaries in chorionic villi. The deoxygenated maternal blood returns to the **uterine veins** and eventually the maternal pulmonary circulation, where carbon dioxide is expelled and fresh oxygen is dissolved in maternal blood for return to the uterine artery. Deoxygenated fetal blood enters the placenta through the **umbilical arteries**. These blood vessels send branches into the chorionic villi where there is a complex anastomosing network of capillaries. In these villi, fetal blood becomes oxygenated and then drains back into the **umbilical vein**. The umbilical vein carrying oxygenated fetal blood shunts by the liver through the **ductus venosus**, empties into the fetal **inferior vena cava**, and enters the right atrium. Before birth, this blood is mostly shunted through the foramen ovale into the left atrium and then into the fetal systemic circulation. Some of this oxygenated blood mixes with deoxygenated blood returning to the right atrium from the superior vena cava and then enters the right ventricle where it is pumped into the pulmonary artery. Most of the blood leaving the right ventricle is shunted away from the lungs into the systemic circulation at the arch of the aorta by way of the **ductus arteriosus**.

Items 232-233

During a squash match, a 35-year-old male experiences sharp pain in his lower back. The next day, he experiences stiffness in his back, complete lack of flexion of the vertebral column due to pain, a dull intense pain in the right buttock and numbness in the lateral surface of the right lower limb. MRI reveals a severe herniated L4-L5 intervertebral disc on the right side.

Choose the **BEST** response.

232. The structure causing the pain in the buttock and numbness in the lower limb is the

    (A)   annulus fibrosus
    (B)   nucleus pulposus
    (C)   ligamentum flavum
    (D)   vertebral arch
    (E)   transverse vertebral process

233. The offending structure is derived from which embryonic structure?

    (A)   notochord
    (B)   intermediate mesoderm
    (C)   dermatome
    (D)   myotome
    (E)   sclerotome

The answers are: **232-B; 233-A**. **Ruptured intervertebral discs** are often caused by a traumatic tearing of the **annulus fibrosus** followed by expulsion of the semi-liquid **nucleus pulposus** so that it traumatizes the nerve roots, causing pain, numbness and possible loss of motor function. Lower back pain is particularly common in humans because we have a vertebral column better suited for quadrupedal locomotion in spite of the fact that we are bipedal. Our erect posture places large compressive forces on the lumbar intervertebral discs.

The **notochord** is a mesodermally derived structure that runs along much of the length of the embryonic body beneath the neural tube. As the vertebral column forms from the sclerotomes, the notochordal component of the vertebral bodies degenerates and disappears. The notochordal component of the intervertebral discs, however, persists in the adult as the nucleus pulposus.

Examine **Figure 2.12** below and then choose the **BEST** response to the items below concerning this photomicrograph. It is a histological preparation of a developing human embryo sectioned through the thoracic level of the body and includes the developing heart (H). Answers may be used once, more than once, or not at all.

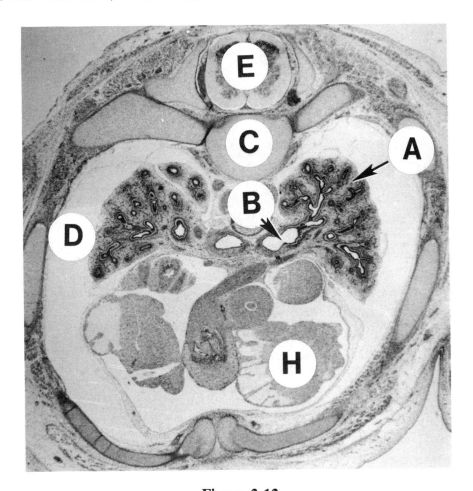

Figure 2.12

234. The embryonic rudiment labeled A gives rise to all of the following structures **EXCEPT**:

   (A)   blood vessels
   (B)   connective tissue
   (C)   pulmonary macrophages
   (D)   visceral pleura
   (E)   lymphatic vessels

235. The embryonic rudiment labeled B gives rise to all of the following structures **EXCEPT**:

   (A)   ciliated cells
   (B)   goblet cells
   (C)   brush cells
   (D)   basal cells
   (E)   chondrocytes

236. The embryonic rudiment labeled C gives rise to which adult structure?

   (A)   neural arch
   (B)   transverse process
   (C)   spinous process
   (D)   nucleus pulposus
   (E)   vertebral body

237. The space labeled D is derived from the _____ and becomes the _____

   (A)   extraembryonic coelom-allantois
   (B)   intraembryonic coelom-peritoneal cavity
   (C)   extraembryonic coelom-diaphragm
   (D)   intraembryonic coelom-pleural cavity
   (E)   septum transversum-diaphragm

238. What is the approximate age of this specimen from time of fertilization?

   (A)   1-3 weeks
   (B)   4-5 weeks
   (C)   6-8 weeks
   (D)   10-12 weeks
   (E)   16-18 weeks

239. The immature organ labeled by A and B will become differentiated enough to be capable of supporting extrauterine life in approximately

   (A)   14 weeks
   (B)   16 weeks
   (C)   18 weeks
   (D)   20 weeks
   (E)   greater than 20 weeks

The answers are: **234-C; 235-E; 236-E; 237-D; 238-C; 239-E**. **Figure 2.12** is a histological section through the developing heart and lungs taken at 6-8 weeks of development. The developing lungs are in the **pseudoglandular stage** of histogenesis which extends from 4 weeks to 15 weeks. During this phase, the trachea, bronchi and bronchioles form. The **canalicular stage** covers 16 weeks to 24 weeks and is a period of formation of terminal bronchioles, respiratory bronchioles and blood vessels. The **saccular stage** extends from 25 weeks to 38 weeks and is a period when many alveoli form. **Type II cells**, producing surfactant, first appear around 28 weeks of development. When large numbers of these cells differentiate, the lungs become functionally mature and the fetus becomes viable in the extrauterine environment. Thus, these lungs will not be functionally mature for more than 20 weeks after the period illustrated in the photomicrograph.

The lungs form from two separate rudiments: the **splanchnic mesoderm** (A) and the **lung buds** (B). The respiratory diverticulum arises as a branch from the foregut at 4 weeks. The respiratory diverticulum grows caudally and branches into left and right lung buds. The lung buds continue to branch and grow into the splanchnic mesoderm. The epithelial components of the respiratory system lining the airways are derived from the respiratory diverticulum. Thus, the epithelial linings of the trachea, bronchi, bronchioles and alveoli are all derived from the respiratory diverticulum. The blood and lymphatic vessels, connective tissue, smooth muscle and cartilage in the remainder of the respiratory system are derived from splanchnic mesoderm. **Pulmonary macrophages**, like all other components of the mononuclear phagocyte system, are derived from bone marrow stem cells. C is a sclerotome-derived **hyaline cartilage** destined to become a vertebral body by endochondral ossification. The intraembryonic coelom is the precursor of the **pleural cavities** (D), pericardial cavity, and peritoneal cavity. The growth of the pleuropericardial membranes and the diaphragm lead to the division of the intraembryonic coelom into these four separate serous cavities. E is the **neural tube**.

Examine the photomicrograph of a developing eye in **Figure 2.13** below. Match the labeled structure with the **MOST** appropriate statement concerning its developmental role in the items below. Answers may be used once, more than once, or not at all.

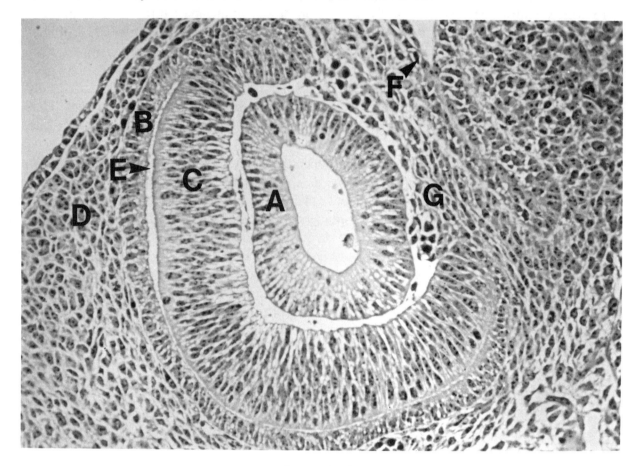

Figure 2.13

240. This structure induces invagination of the optic vesicle.

241. This structure is crucially involved in retinal detachment secondary to head trauma.

242. This structure forms phagocytic cells associated with rod outer segments.

243. This structure forms the corneal epithelium.

244. This structure forms the corneal endothelium and anterior chamber.

ANSWERS AND TUTORIAL ON ITEMS 240-244

The answers are: **240-A; 241-E; 242-B; 243-F; 244-G**. **Figure 2.13** is a histological section of a developing mouse eye. It is approximately equivalent to a developing human eye at about 5 weeks of development. The **lens vesicle** (A) is derived from an invagination of the surface ectoderm. It is induced by the optic vesicle and in turn, induces the invagination of the optic vesicle to form an optic cup. The optic cup has two distinct layers, an outer **pigmented retinal epithelium** (B) and an inner **neural retinal epithelium** (C). The former forms the simple cuboidal epithelium of the definitive pigmented retina. The latter forms the photosensitive portion of the retina, complete with rods, cones, bipolar cells, and ganglion cells which project their axons into the optic stalk, eventually forming the optic nerve. **Posterior head mesenchymal cells** (D) condense around the outer layer of the optic cup and eventually form the choroid layer and the sclera. The **intraretinal space** (E) is a remnant of the lumen of the central nervous system and earlier was in direct communication with the third brain ventricle. It is a potential space in the adult eye where the apical, nonadhesive layers of the pigmented retina and neural retina come in contact. These two layers are loosely bound to each other and can separate (e.g., from a blow to the head) leading to retinal detachment. The **surface ectoderm** (F) anterior to the lens forms the corneal epithelium. **Anterior head mesenchymal cells** (G) contribute to the corneal stroma and corneal endothelium (the name used for this structure in definitive histology textbooks). The corneal endothelium is also called corneal mesothelium, the name used in embryology textbooks. This name does not seem appropriate because mesothelium is usually reserved for the mesodermally derived simple squamous epithelium lining serous body cavities. The anterior chamber of the eye is directly connected to the cardiovascular system via the canal of Schlemm. Therefore, the name corneal endothelium seems preferable. The anterior chamber of the eye also forms from fusion of small vesicles in the mesenchyme posterior to the cornea into a cleft-like space, much like blood vessels, reinforcing the use of the term corneal endothelium.

Examine the labeled drawing of an adult ear in **Figure 2.14** below. Match the statements below on ear development with the **MOST** appropriate labeled structure. Answers may be used once, more than once, or not at all.

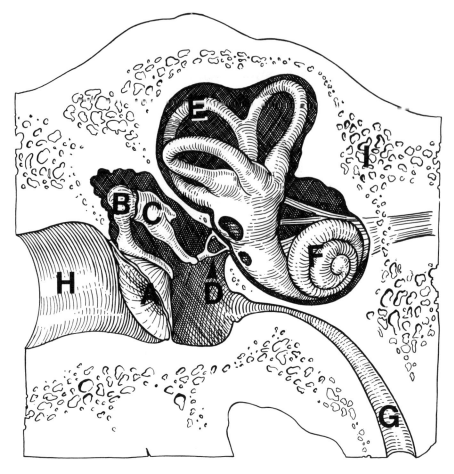

Figure 2.14

245. This structure is formed from the utricular portion of the otocyst.

246. This structure is formed from the saccular portion of the otocyst.

247. This structure is formed from the first pharyngeal pouch.

248. This structure is formed from the first pharyngeal groove.

249. This structure is formed from the otic capsule and will become dense bone.

250. This structure is formed from second pharyngeal arch mesenchyme.

ANSWERS AND TUTORIAL ON ITEMS 245-250

The answers are: **245-E; 246-F; 247-G; 248-H; 249-I; 250-D**. **Figure 2.14** is a diagram of the human middle and inner ear. The **tympanic membrane** (A) is a derivative of the first pharyngeal membrane which lies between the first pharyngeal groove [**external auditory meatus** (H) precursor] and the first pharyngeal pouch [**auditory** or eustachian **tube** (G) precursor].

The **malleus** (B), **incus** (C) and **stapes** (D) are the three middle ear ossicles. They conduct vibrations from the tympanic membrane to the oval window. The malleus and incus form in the first pharyngeal arch. The stapes forms in the second pharyngeal arch.

The **bony labyrinth** (I) is a cavity within the petrous temporal bone. It contains the membranous labyrinth which is derived from the **otocyst**. The otocyst is formed by invagination of surface ectoderm and undergoes a shape change to form a **utricular portion** and a **saccular portion**. The utricular portion forms the **semicircular ducts** (E), endolymphatic duct, and the utricle. The saccular portion forms the saccule and the **cochlear duct** (F).

CHAPTER III

GROSS ANATOMY

Items 251-254

A 21-year-old man falls through a window and suffers a deep gash in the posterolateral neck on the left. Examination reveals that the level of the left shoulder is lower than that of the right shoulder, and that the patient has difficulty in shrugging the left shoulder against resistance. There is no increase in the tone of the muscle underlying the medial part of the upper border of the left shoulder when the patient attempts to shrug the left shoulder.

Choose the **BEST** response.

251. Which nerve or part of the brachial plexus has been cut as demonstrated by the physical exam?

    (A) axillary nerve
    (B) spinal part of the accessory nerve
    (C) dorsal scapular nerve
    (D) suprascapular nerve
    (E) upper trunk of the brachial plexus

252. Which of the following active movements will also prove difficult for the patient as suggested by the physical exam?

    (A) flexing the left arm 60°
    (B) extending the left arm 60°
    (C) abducting the left arm more than 90°
    (D) internally rotating the left arm
    (E) externally rotating the left arm

253. A deep gash in the posterolateral aspect of the neck may result in a loss of sensation in any of the following areas **EXCEPT**:

    (A) skin of the anterior aspect of the neck
    (B) skin overlying the clavicle
    (C) skin overlying the angle of the mandible
    (D) skin of the lobule of the ear
    (E) skin of the chin

254. A deep gash in the posterior triangle of the neck can cut the

    (A)   common carotid artery
    (B)   external carotid artery
    (C)   internal carotid artery
    (D)   external jugular vein
    (E)   internal jugular vein

ANSWERS AND TUTORIAL ON ITEMS 251-254

The answers are: **251-B; 252-C; 253-E; 254-D**. Flaccidity of the muscle mass underlying the medial part of the upper border of the shoulder indicates **trapezius palsy** which suggests a cut through the spinal part of the **accessory nerve** in the posterior triangle of the neck. A deep gash in the posterior triangle of the neck may cut nerves and blood vessels such as the spinal part of the accessory nerve, branches of the cervical plexus, the supraclavicular parts of the brachial plexus, and the external jugular vein. The posterior triangle of the neck is bordered anteriorly by the posterior border of **sternocleidomastoid** (S), posteriorly by the anterior border of **trapezius** (T), and inferiorly by the middle third of the **clavicle** (C) (**Figure 3.1**).

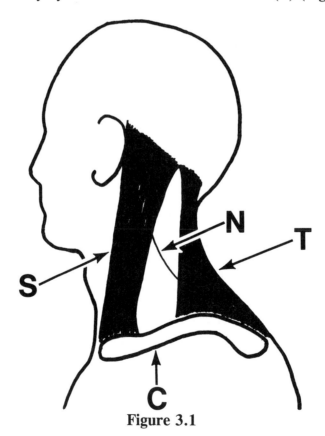

Figure 3.1

The spinal part of the accessory nerve arises from fibers that emerge from spinal cord segments C1 through C5. The fibers form a trunk within the vertebral canal that first ascends into the cranial cavity through the foramen magnum and then descends into the neck after exiting the skull through the jugular foramen. The spinal part of the accessory nerve pierces and innervates sternocleidomastoid, crosses the posterior triangle of the neck, and finally passes deep to trapezius which it innervates. The spinal part of the accessory nerve (N) is susceptible to injury along its descent across the posterior triangle of the neck, for here it lies covered only by skin, superficial fascia and the investing layer of deep cervical fascia (**Figure 3.1**).

Trapezius is the chief muscle that supports the scapula and clavicle from the axial skeleton. It is responsible for elevating the shoulders as in shrugging. Trapezius is also a prime mover for lateral rotation of the scapula, the movement by which the clavicle rotates at the sternoclavicular joint and the scapula rotates at the acromioclavicular joint in such a fashion that the inferior angle of the scapula moves laterally and upward. Abduction of the arm above the shoulder requires lateral rotation of the scapula. Consequently, loss of innervation to trapezius results in a lowering of the shoulder and weakness in either shrugging or abducting the arm above the shoulder. Isolated trapezius palsy also results in flaring of the vertebral border and inferior angle of the scapula. Abduction of the arm against resistance accentuates the flaring, but flexion of the arm minimizes it.

The cutaneous branches of the **cervical plexus** all emerge around the posterior border of sternocleidomastoid en route to their areas of cutaneous innervation. The **transverse cervical nerve** (C2,3) provides general sensory innervation for almost all the skin overlying the anterior triangle of the neck (region TC in **Figure 3.2**). The **supraclavicular nerves** (C3,4) provide sensory innervation for the skin overlying the top of the shoulder (in particular that overlying the

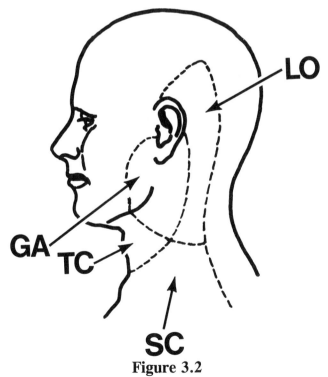

Figure 3.2

113

clavicle) (region SC in **Figure 3.2**). The **great auricular nerve** (C2,3) provides sensory innervation for the skin overlying the angle of the mandible, the lower part of the parotid gland, the mastoid process, and almost all of the auricle (including the lobule) (region GA in **Figure 3.2**). The **lesser occipital nerve** (C2) provides sensory innervation for the strip of the scalp immediately posterior to the auricle (region LO in **Figure 3.2**). A branch of the **mandibular division of the trigeminal nerve** provides sensory innervation for the skin of the chin.

The **external jugular vein** descends across the lower part of the posterior triangle of the neck before passing through the investing layer of deep cervical fascia to join the subclavian vein. The investing layer of deep cervical fascia is attached to the outer surface of the vein at the site where the vein pierces the fascia. This fascial attachment promotes patency of the vein. Consequently, if the external jugular vein is cut anywhere above its attachment to the investing layer of deep cervical fascia in the posterior triangle of the neck, there is the risk that a pulmonary embolism will occur as a result of air being sucked into the vein during inspiration.

Items 255-257

An 18-year-old man injures the right shoulder from a downward blow on the point of the shoulder. The acromion of the scapula lies anteroinferior to the lateral end of the clavicle. There is tenderness in the region between the acromion and the lateral end of the clavicle and pain when abducting the right arm up to or above the level of the shoulder. Anteroposterior (AP) radiographs show that the acromioclavicular and coracoclavicular spaces in the right shoulder are each more than 50% wider than the corresponding spaces in the left shoulder.

Choose the **BEST** response.

255.   Which bony structure lies **DIRECTLY** beneath the skin at the point of the shoulder?

   (A)   acromion of the scapula
   (B)   coracoid process of the scapula
   (C)   spine of the scapula
   (D)   superior angle of the scapula
   (E)   head of the humerus

256. The AP radiographs of the shoulders indicate which of the following ligaments is significantly ruptured in the right shoulder?

    (A)   costoclavicular ligament
    (B)   coracoacromial ligament
    (C)   coracohumeral ligament
    (D)   coracoclavicular ligament
    (E)   suprascapular ligament

257. Which injury is **MOST** indicated by the history, physical exam, and radiographs?

    (A)   acromioclavicular joint sprain
    (B)   acromioclavicular joint subluxation
    (C)   acromioclavicular joint dislocation
    (D)   shoulder joint dislocation
    (E)   sternoclavicular joint dislocation

ANSWERS AND TUTORIAL ON ITEMS 255-257

The answers are: **255-A; 256-D; 257-C**. The point of the shoulder is the lateral-most limit of the shoulder. The acromion of the scapula lies directly beneath the skin here and thus gives the point of the shoulder its shape. Downward blows on the point of the shoulder strain the fibrous structures that suspend the scapula from the clavicle, in particular, the capsule of the **acromioclavicular joint** (AC) and the **coracoclavicular ligament** (CL) (**Figure 3.3**). In this case, the anteroinferior displacement of the acromion indicates dislocation of the acromioclavicular joint (a Grade III shoulder separation), and the radiographs confirm the diagnosis. Injuries of the acromioclavicular joint are called **shoulder separations**. Tenderness over the acromioclavicular joint is common. Abduction of the arm beyond 90° is frequently painful.

The severity of a shoulder separation is assessed by comparing the widths of the acromioclavicular and coracoclavicular spaces in an AP radiograph of the injured shoulder with the widths of the corresponding spaces of the uninjured shoulder. The acromioclavicular space is the radiolucent space between the acromion and the lateral end of the clavicle and marks the apposed articular cartilages in the acromioclavicular joint. The coracoclavicular space is the radiolucent space between the coracoid process of the scapula and the clavicle above and marks the coracoclavicular ligament. The coracoclavicular ligament is the principal ligamentous structure that suspends the scapula from the clavicle.

A simple sprain of the acromioclavicular joint capsule is called a **Grade I** shoulder separation. In such an injury, the capsule sustains minimal tearing, and an AP radiograph of the injured shoulder shows normal acromioclavicular and coracoclavicular spaces without deformity.

A subluxation (partial dislocation) of the acromioclavicular joint is called a **Grade II** shoulder separation. It results from a significant rupture of the acromioclavicular joint capsule. An AP radiograph of the injured shoulder shows an acromioclavicular space whose width is at least 50% greater than that of the uninjured shoulder. Inspection of the injured shoulder generally shows the lateral end of the clavicle a step above the acromion.

A dislocation of the acromioclavicular joint is called a **Grade III** shoulder separation. It occurs when both the acromioclavicular joint capsule and the coracoclavicular ligament are significantly ruptured. An AP radiograph of the injured shoulder shows acromioclavicular and coracoclavicular spaces at least 50% wider than those of the uninjured shoulder. Inspection of the injured shoulder commonly shows the acromion displaced anteroinferiorly to the lateral end of the clavicle.

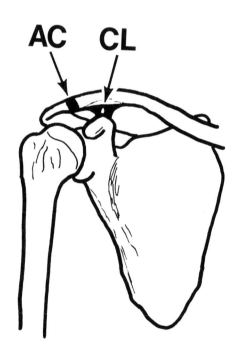

Figure 3.3

Figure 3.4 is a diagram of the **brachial plexus**. The anterior rami of C5, C6, C7, C8 and T1 form the roots of the plexus. The **middle cervical ganglion** (MCG) of the sympathetic chain communicates with the C5 and C6 roots, the **lower cervical ganglion** (LCG) communicates with the C7 and C8 roots, and the **first thoracic ganglion** (1TG) communicates with the T1 root. The C5 and C6 roots unite to form the **upper trunk** (UT), the C7 root extends to become the **middle trunk** (MT), and the C8 and T1 roots unite to form the **lower trunk** (LT) of the plexus. The anterior divisions of the upper and middle trunks unite to form the **lateral cord** (LC), the posterior divisions of all three trunks unite to form the **posterior cord** (PC), and the anterior division of the lower trunk extends to become the **medial cord** (MC) of the plexus.

    Figure 3.5 displays 10 sites in the brachial plexus at which injury can produce serious losses of muscle action and skin sensation in the upper limb.

(A) C5 root proximal to the sympathetic chain
(B) C5 root distal to the sympathetic chain
(C) upper trunk
(D) lateral cord
(E) middle trunk
(F) posterior cord
(G) T1 root proximal to the sympathetic chain
(H) T1 root distal to the sympathetic chain
(I) lower trunk
(J) medial cord

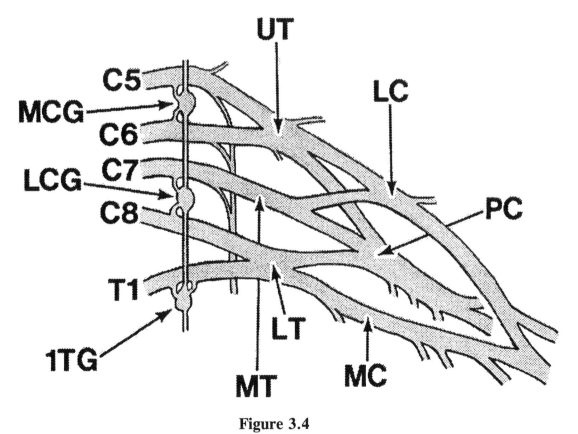

Figure 3.4

117

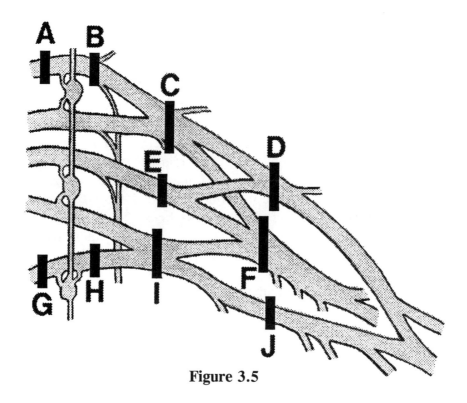

Figure 3.5

In answering Items 258-263, assume that the brachial plexus has been injured at one of the sites displayed in **Figure 3.5**.

Choose the **BEST** response.

258. Identify the **ONLY** site at which a severe injury could

    (i)   completely paralyze the muscles that initiate abduction of the arm from the anatomic position,

    (ii)   cause the biceps brachii deep tendon reflex to be absent, and

    (iii)   markedly diminish sensation on the lateral aspect of the arm and forearm.

259. Identify the **ONLY** site at which a severe injury could

    (i)   completely paralyze the prime mover of opposition of the thumb,

    (ii)   completely paralyze the muscles that abduct and adduct the fingers, and

    (iii)   markedly diminish the triceps brachii deep tendon reflex.

260. There are two sites displayed in **Figure 3.5** at which a severe injury could markedly diminish sensation on the medial aspect of the forearm and arm. Identify the **MORE PROXIMAL** site.

118

261. Identify the **ONLY** site at which a severe injury could cause the triceps brachii deep tendon reflex to be absent.

262. Identify the **ONLY** site at which a severe injury could

   (i)   partially paralyze the muscles that abduct and adduct the fingers,
   (ii)   partially paralyze the prime mover of opposition of the thumb, and
   (iii) cause the upper eyelid to droop.

263. Identify the **ONLY** site at which a severe injury would diminish sensation at the tip of the middle finger more markedly than it diminishes sensation at the tips of the thumb and little finger.

ANSWERS AND TUTORIAL ON ITEMS 258-263

The answers are: **258-C; 259-I; 260-I; 261-F; 262-G; 263-E**. Severe traction is the mechanism by which the brachial plexus is commonly injured. **Upper brachial plexus injuries**: Traction injuries of the upper parts of the brachial plexus typically involve the C5 and C6 roots and/or upper trunk of the plexus. Upper plexus traction injuries thus chiefly affect those upper limb movements whose prime movers are muscles innervated exclusively by C5 and C6 nerve fibers (supraspinatus, infraspinatus, teres minor, deltoid, biceps brachii, and supinator) or predominantly by C5 and C6 nerve fibers (brachialis and brachioradialis). The cutaneous sensory losses associated with upper plexus traction injuries chiefly involve the lateral aspect of the arm and forearm and the palmar and dorsal surfaces of the thumb (**Figures 3.6A** and **3.6B**). **Figures 3.6A** and **3.6B** show, respectively, the dermatomes on the anterior and posterior surfaces of the upper limb.

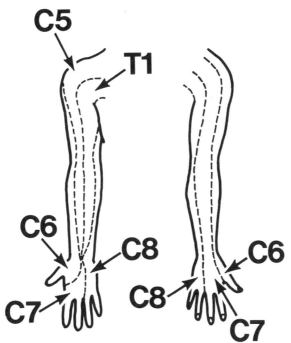

Figure 3.6A and B

119

Item 258 highlights some of the most important motor and sensory deficits that can result from a severe traction injury to the **upper trunk of the brachial plexus**. A severe injury to the upper trunk can (i) completely paralyze the muscles that initiate abduction of the arm from the anatomic position, (ii) completely paralyze the muscles that supinate the forearm, (iii) almost completely paralyze the muscles that flex the forearm, and (iv) markedly diminish sensation on the lateral aspects of the arm and forearm and the palmar and dorsal surfaces of the thumb.

Supraspinatus and **deltoid** are the muscles that initiate abduction of the arm from the anatomic position. Supraspinatus is innervated by the suprascapular nerve (SN), which is a branch of the upper trunk (**Figure 3.7**). Deltoid is innervated by the axillary nerve (AN), which is one of the two terminal branches of the posterior cord of the brachial plexus (**Figure 3.7**). The solid, black tracings in **Figure 3.7** represent the C5 and C6 nerve fibers in the axillary nerve that innervate deltoid (and also teres minor). The fibers enter the plexus via the C5 and C6 roots and then extend through the upper trunk and posterior cord before exiting the plexus via the axillary nerve.

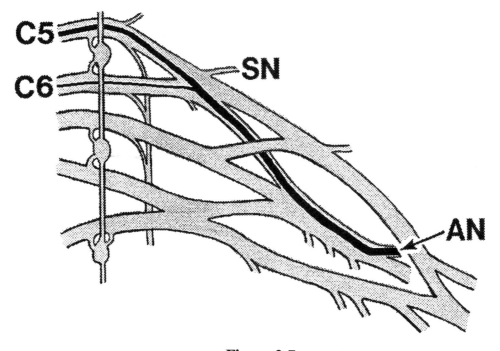

Figure 3.7

Biceps brachii is a chief flexor and supinator of the forearm. Biceps brachii is innervated by the musculocutaneous nerve (MUN), which is a major branch of the lateral cord of the brachial plexus (**Figure 3.8**). The solid, black tracings in **Figure 3.8** represent the C5 and C6 nerve fibers that innervate biceps brachii. The fibers enter the plexus via the C5 and C6 roots and then extend through the upper trunk and lateral cord before exiting the plexus via the musculocutaneous nerve. The biceps brachii deep tendon reflex is a reflex whose afferent (sensory) nerve fibers enter the spinal cord at the C5 and C6 levels and whose efferent (motor) nerve fibers exit the spinal cord at the C5 and C6 levels.

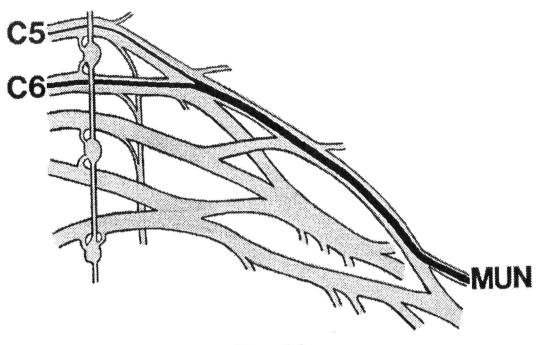

Figure 3.8

Upper plexus traction injuries that profoundly paralyze supraspinatus, deltoid and biceps brachii tend to cause the affected upper limb to hang by the side of the body with the forearm pronated. The arm hangs by the side of the body because of the inability or weakened ability to abduct the arm at the shoulder joint. The forearm tends to be extended because the major flexors of the forearm (biceps brachii and brachialis) are profoundly paralyzed (brachialis receives most of its nerve fibers from the C5 and C6 levels of the spinal cord). The forearm tends to be pronated because both supinators of the forearm (biceps brachii and supinator) are profoundly paralyzed (supinator receives all its motor nerve fibers from the C5 and C6 levels of the spinal cord). Because the upper limb, under these conditions, exhibits a position similar to that assumed by a waiter awaiting a tip, the paralysis is frequently described as a 'waiter's tip palsy.' The paralysis may also referred to as Erb's palsy.

Lower brachial plexus injuries: Traction injuries of the lower parts of the brachial plexus typically involve the C8 and T1 roots and/or lower trunk of the plexus. Lower plexus traction injuries thus chiefly affect those upper limb movements whose prime movers are muscles innervated either exclusively or predominantly by C8 and T1 fibers (flexor carpi ulnaris, flexor digitorum superficialis, flexor digitorum profundus, flexor pollicis longus, pronator quadratus, extensor carpi ulnaris, abductor pollicis longus, extensor pollicis brevis, extensor pollicis longus, extensor indicis, and all the intrinsic muscles of the hand). In effect, lower plexus traction injuries can affect virtually all movements of the hand and its digits. The cutaneous sensory losses associated with lower plexus traction injuries chiefly involve the medial aspect of the arm and forearm and the palmar and dorsal surfaces of the ring and little fingers (**Figures 3.6A** and **3.6B**).

Items 259 and 260 highlight some of the most important motor and sensory deficits that can result from a severe traction injury to the **lower trunk of the brachial plexus**. A severe injury to the lower trunk can (i) completely paralyze the prime mover of opposition of the thumb, (ii) completely paralyze the muscles that abduct and adduct the fingers, (iii) markedly weaken the muscle that extends the forearm, and (iv) markedly diminish sensation on the medial aspect of the arm and forearm and the palmar and dorsal surfaces of the ring and little fingers.

Opposition of the thumb is the movement by which the tip of the thumb is brought into contact with the tips of the fingers. **Opponens pollicis**, a muscle of the thenar eminence, is the prime mover for opposition of the thumb. Opponens pollicis is innervated by the median nerve (MEN), which is formed by the union of fibers from both the medial and lateral cords of the brachial plexus (**Figure 3.9**). All the motor nerve fibers that innervate opponens pollicis (as well as the other two muscles of the thenar eminence, abductor pollicis brevis and flexor pollicis brevis) arise from the C8 and T1 levels of the spinal cord. The majority of these fibers arise from the C8 level. The solid, black tracings in **Figure 3.9** represent the C8 and T1 nerve fibers that innervate the muscles of the thenar eminence; the fibers enter the plexus via the C8 and T1 roots and then extend through the lower trunk and medial cord before exiting the plexus via the median nerve.

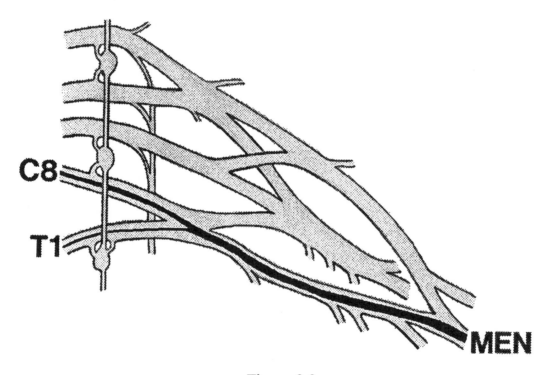

Figure 3.9

The **palmar** and **dorsal interossei** and **abductor digiti minimi** (a muscle of the hypothenar eminence) are the abductors and adductors of the fingers. The palmar and dorsal interossei and abductor digiti minimi are all innervated by the deep branch of the ulnar nerve, and the ulnar nerve (UN) is one of the major branches of the medial cord of the brachial plexus (**Figure 3.10**). All the motor nerve fibers that innervate these muscles arise from the C8 and T1 levels of the spinal cord. The majority of these fibers arise from the T1 level. The solid, black tracings in **Figure 3.10** represent the C8 and T1 nerve fibers that innervate the palmar and dorsal interossei and abductor digiti minimi. The fibers enter the plexus via the C8 and T1 roots and then extend through the lower trunk and medial cord before exiting the plexus via the ulnar nerve.

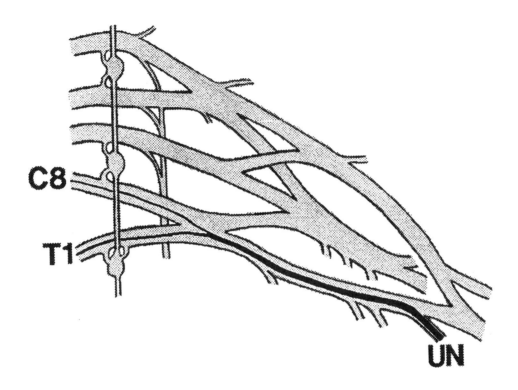

Figure 3.10

Triceps brachii is the extensor of the forearm. Triceps brachii is innervated by the radial nerve (RN), one of the two terminal branches of the posterior cord of the brachial plexus (**Figure 3.11**). The motor nerve fibers that innervate triceps brachii arise from the C6, C7, and C8 levels of the spinal cord. The majority of these fibers arise from the C7 and C8 levels. The solid, black tracings in **Figure 3.11** represent the C6, C7, and C8 nerve fibers that innervate triceps brachii; the fibers enter the plexus via the C6, C7, and C8 roots, pass through the upper, middle and lower trunks and then finally extend through the posterior cord before exiting the plexus via the radial nerve. The triceps brachii deep tendon reflex is a reflex whose afferent (sensory) nerve fibers enter the spinal cord at primarily the C7 and C8 levels and whose efferent (motor) nerve fibers exit the spinal cord at primarily the C7 and C8 levels.

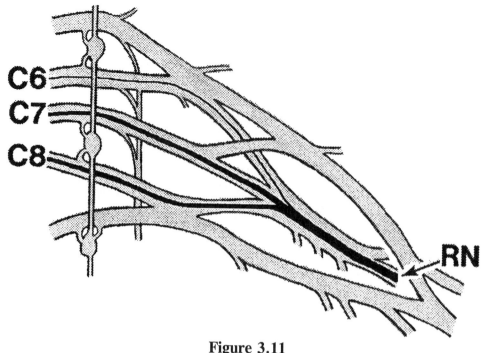

Figure 3.11

The medial cutaneous nerve of the arm (MCNA) and the medial cutaneous nerve of the forearm (MCNF) are the nerves which provide cutaneous innervation for the medial aspect of, respectively, the arm and forearm (**Figure 3.12**). Both nerves transmit sensory nerve fibers that project to the C8 and T1 levels of the spinal cord. With respect to Item 260, I and J are the two sites displayed in **Figure 3.5** at which a severe injury could markedly diminish sensation on the medial aspect of the forearm and arm. This is because I and J are the only sites displayed in **Figure 3.5** at which a severe injury would affect both the C8 and T1 sensory nerve fibers in the medial cutaneous nerves of the arm and forearm.

Injury to the **posterior cord**: The answer to Item 261 is F because F is the only site in **Figure 3.5** which transmits all the C6, C7, and C8 nerve fibers to triceps brachii. Brachial plexus injuries involving the **sympathetic chain**: Severe traction injuries of the lower parts of the brachial plexus can also affect sympathetic innervation of tissues in the head. The preganglionic sympathetic fibers involved in the sympathetic innervation of tissues in the head arise, for the most part, from the T1, T2, and T3 levels of the spinal cord. The solid black tracing in **Figure 3.12** shows how the preganglionic sympathetic fibers that arise from the T1 level of the spinal cord extend from the T1 root of the brachial plexus through the white ramus communicans (WRC) and the first thoracic ganglion (1TG) before ascending the sympathetic chain to the superior cervical ganglion (the superior cervical ganglion is not shown in **Figure 3.12**). In the superior cervical ganglion, the preganglionic sympathetic fibers synapse with postganglionic sympathetic neurons; the fibers that arise from these postganglionic sympathetic neurons provide sympathetic innervation to tissues of the head and upper neck.

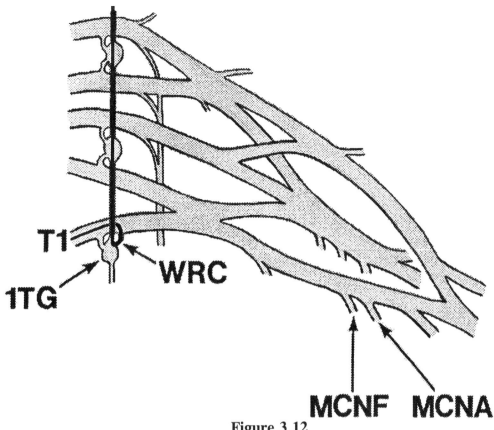

Figure 3.12

Significant injury to the preganglionic sympathetic fibers that are involved in the sympathetic innervation of tissues in the head produces three deficits collectively referred to as **Horner's syndrome**. The three deficits of **Horner's syndrome** are **ptosis** (a drooping upper eyelid), **miosis** (a constricted pupil) and **anhydrosis** (an absence of sweating on the affected side of the head). **Levator palpebrae superioris**, the muscle responsible for raising the upper eyelid, consists of both skeletal muscle and smooth muscle fibers. The oculomotor nerve innervates the skeletal muscle fibers, and sympathetic fibers innervate the smooth muscle fibers. Paralysis of either set of muscle fibers results in drooping of the upper eyelid. Therefore, of the sites indicated in **Figure 3.5**, only G is the site at which injury could result in drooping of the upper eyelid. As previously discussed, injury at site G can also partially paralyze opponens pollicis and the muscles that abduct and adduct the fingers.

Injury to the **middle trunk**: With respect to Item 263, reference to **Figures 3.6A** and **3.6B** shows that the skin of the thumb is part of the C6 dermatome, that of the middle finger part of the C7 dermatome, and that of the little finger part of the C8 dermatome. Recall that three spinal nerves typically provide cutaneous innervation in each of the dermatomes of the body: the dermatome's spinal nerve is the chief source of the cutaneous innervation, and the spinal nerves for the adjacent dermatomes provide the remainder of the cutaneous innervation. For example, in the skin of the middle finger, C7 sensory fibers are the chief source of cutaneous innervation, and C6 and C8 sensory fibers provide the remainder of the cutaneous innervation. E is the only site displayed in **Figure 3.5** at which a severe injury would damage C7 but neither C6 nor C8 sensory nerve fibers.

A 19-year-old woman has a painful right shoulder one day after playing basketball. She fell twice during the game, each time using the right upper limb to protect the body against impact with the floor. The right shoulder is not obviously deformed but there is tenderness between the acromion of the scapula and the greater tuberosity of the humerus. Abduction of the arm from the anatomic position against resistance is painful. Although the patient can actively abduct the right arm from 0 to 60° and from 120 to 180°, pain accompanies active and passive abduction from 60 to 120°.

Choose the **BEST** response.

264. Which of the following injuries is **MOST LIKELY** given the history and physical exam?

    (A)   shoulder joint dislocation
    (B)   tear of the deltoid muscle
    (C)   fracture of the clavicle
    (D)   incomplete tear of the supraspinatus tendon
    (E)   complete tear of the supraspinatus tendon

265. Each of the following statements concerning arm abduction through the 60 to 120° arc is correct **EXCEPT**:

    (A)   Movement through the arc involves abduction of the humerus at the shoulder joint.
    (B)   Movement through the arc involves lateral rotation of the scapula at the acromioclavicular joint.
    (C)   The muscles of the rotator cuff act as prime movers.
    (D)   Serratus anterior and trapezius act as prime movers.
    (E)   The supraspinatus tendon and subacromial bursa are pulled proximally beneath the acromion of the scapula.

266. Each of the following muscles contributes to the rotator cuff of the shoulder joint **EXCEPT**:

    (A)   teres minor
    (B)   teres major
    (C)   supraspinatus
    (D)   infraspinatus
    (E)   subscapularis

ANSWERS AND TUTORIAL ON ITEMS 264-266

The answers are: **264-D; 265-C; 266-B**. Painful arm abduction that extends in an ac from about 60 to 120° suggests a lesion of the **supraspinatus tendon** of insertion or inflammation of the **subacromial bursa**. The history, presence of tenderness between the acromion and greater tuberosity, and pain upon abduction of the arm from the anatomic position against resistance, all suggest an incomplete rupture of the supraspinatus tendon.

Supraspinatus, infraspinatus, teres minor, and **subscapularis** all originate from the scapula and insert onto the fibrous capsule of the shoulder joint and either the greater or lesser tuberosity of the humerus. The tendons of these four muscles form the **rotator cuff** (so named because infraspinatus and teres minor are external rotators of the arm and subscapularis is an internal rotator). The muscles of the rotator cuff are not powerful movers of the arm. However, when powerful muscles (such as deltoid, pectoralis major, teres major, and latissimus dorsi) move the arm at the shoulder joint, the muscles of the rotator cuff are dynamic stabilizers of the humeral head in the glenoid fossa of the scapula.

During abduction and flexion of the arm, the **supraspinatus tendon** (T) and the **subacromial bursa** (B) are subject to compression and friction between the head of the humerus (H) and the overlying coracoacromial ligament and acromion (A) (**Figure 3.13**). Repetitive application of these potentially disruptive forces can lead to incomplete tear of the supraspinatus tendon, supraspinatus tendinitis, calcified depositions in the supraspinatus tendon, or subacromial bursitis. Arm abduction with any of these lesions is characteristically painless from 0 to 60°, painful from 60 to 120°, and then painless again from 120 to 180°. The intermediate arc is painful because the injured supraspinatus tendon or the inflamed subacromial bursa is pulled proximally and compressed beneath the acromion and/or coracoacromial ligament.

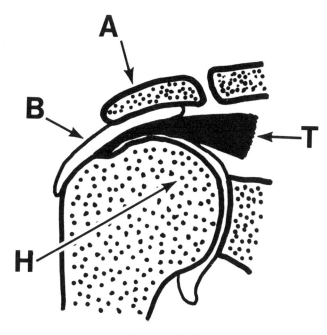

Figure 3.13

Arm abduction involves movements at the sternoclavicular, acromioclavicular, and shoulder joints. Upward rotation of the clavicle at the sternoclavicular joint in combination with upward and outward rotation of the scapula at the acromioclavicular joint produce lateral rotation of the scapula. Upward rotation of the humerus occurs at the shoulder joint. The concerted movements at the three joints produce arm abduction. Upward rotation of the humerus at the shoulder joint contributes 2° abduction for every 1° provided by lateral rotation of the scapula. Supraspinatus and deltoid are the prime movers for initiation of abduction from the anatomic position. For abduction beyond 15°, deltoid is the prime mover for upward rotation of the humerus at the shoulder joint, and serratus anterior and trapezius are the prime movers for lateral rotation of the scapula.

Items 267-269

A 51-year-old man suffers an injury to the right shoulder during an automobile accident. An AP radiograph of the right shoulder reveals an anterior shoulder dislocation in which the head of the humerus lies in a subglenoid position (**Figure 3.14**).

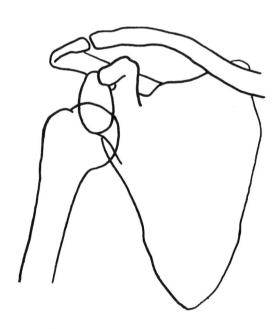

Figure 3.14

Choose the **BEST** response.

267. Which nerve is **MOST** likely to be injured by the inferior displacement of the humeral head?

    (A)   axillary nerve
    (B)   median nerve
    (C)   musculocutaneous nerve
    (D)   radial nerve
    (E)   ulnar nerve

268. If the nerve **MOST** likely to be injured by the inferior displacement of the humeral head is indeed injured, which motor or sensory deficit may be observed following reduction of the dislocation?

    (A)   Weakness in extending the forearm at the elbow against resistance.
    (B)   Weakness in flexing the forearm at the elbow against resistance.
    (C)   Partial loss of sensation on the medial aspect of the upper arm.
    (D)   Partial loss of sensation on the lateral aspect of the upper arm.
    (E)   Weakness in pronating the forearm at the radioulnar joints against resistance.

269. Which of the following arteries passes **DIRECTLY** inferior to the shoulder joint capsule?

    (A)   thoracoacromial trunk
    (B)   anterior circumflex humeral artery
    (C)   posterior circumflex humeral artery
    (D)   lateral thoracic artery
    (E)   subscapular artery

ANSWERS AND TUTORIAL ON ITEMS 267-269

The answers are: **267-A; 268-D; 269-C**. As previously discussed in the tutorial for Items 258-263, the **axillary nerve** (AN) arises from the posterior cord (PC) of the brachial plexus (**Figures 3.7** and **3.15**). The axillary nerve extends toward the posterior part of the upper arm by passing posteriorly through the **quadrangular space** (where it accompanies the posterior circumflex humeral artery, a branch of the third part of the axillary artery). The quadrangular space is bordered medially by the long head of triceps, laterally by the surgical neck (SN) of the humerus, inferiorly by teres major, and superiorly by subscapularis, the fibrous capsule of the shoulder joint (SJ), and teres minor (**Figure 3.15**). The close relation of the axillary nerve to the inferior aspect of the shoulder joint capsule in the quadrangular space renders the axillary nerve especially susceptible to injury from shoulder dislocations in which the humeral head is inferiorly displaced. The close relation of the axillary nerve to the surgical neck of the humerus in the quadrangular space renders the axillary nerve especially susceptible to injury from fractures of the surgical neck.

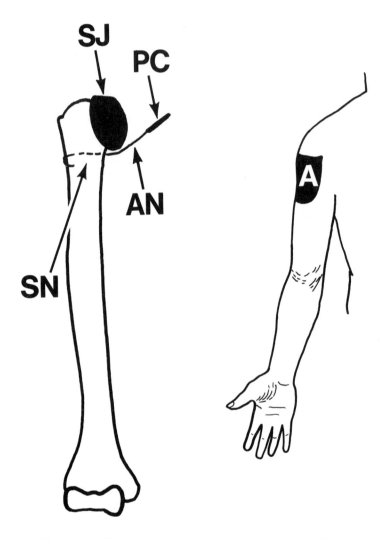

Figure 3.15   **Figure 3.16**

Upon passing through the quadrangular space, the axillary nerve gives rise to the branches which innervate **teres minor** and **deltoid**. The axillary nerve also gives rise to the upper lateral cutaneous nerve of the arm. The cutaneous area (A) supplied by this nerve includes

130

the skin overlying the lower half of deltoid (**Figure 3.16**). The most important motor deficit that can result from injury to the axillary nerve is partial or complete loss of the actions of deltoid. Injury to the axillary nerve may result in sensory deficits in the cutaneous area supplied by the upper lateral cutaneous nerve of the arm.

Items 270-272

Following an automobile accident, radiographs reveal that a 52-year-old woman has sustained an oblique fracture through the midshaft of the humerus.

Choose the **BEST** response.

270.   Which nerve is **MOST** likely to be injured by the midshaft fracture of the humerus?

    (A)   axillary nerve
    (B)   median nerve
    (C)   musculocutaneous nerve
    (D)   radial nerve
    (E)   ulnar nerve

271.   If the nerve **MOST** likely to be injured by the midshaft fracture of the humerus is injured, weakness in all of the following motor functions may be observed after reduction of the fracture **EXCEPT**:

    (A)   extending the hand at the wrist against resistance
    (B)   flexing the hand at the wrist against resistance
    (C)   abducting the hand at the wrist against resistance
    (D)   adducting the hand at the wrist against resistance
    (E)   supinating the forearm against resistance

272.   Each of the following muscles is a major abductor or adductor of the hand **EXCEPT**:

    (A)   brachioradialis
    (B)   extensor carpi ulnaris
    (C)   flexor carpi radialis
    (D)   extensor carpi radialis longus
    (E)   extensor carpi radialis brevis

ANSWERS AND TUTORIAL ON ITEMS 270-272

The answers are: **270-D; 271-B; 272-A**. As previously discussed in the tutorial for Items 258-263, the **radial nerve** (RN) arises from the posterior cord (PC) of the brachial plexus (**Figures 3.11** and **17**). As the radial nerve extends through the midregion of the arm (alongside the deep brachial artery, a branch of the brachial artery), both the radial nerve and deep brachial artery lie against the spiral groove of the shaft of the humerus, rendering the radial nerve especially susceptible to injury from fractures of the midshaft of the humerus.

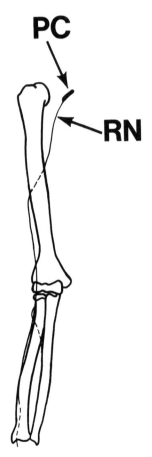

Figure 3.17

Injury to the radial nerve along its course beside the spiral groove of the humerus may cause partial denervation of triceps brachii and partial or complete denervation of any of the forearm muscles innervated by either the radial nerve (brachioradialis and extensor carpi radialis longus) or its branches (supinator, extensor carpi radialis brevis, extensor carpi ulnaris, abductor pollicis longus, extensor pollicis brevis, extensor pollicis longus, extensor digitorum, extensor indicis, and extensor digiti minimi). Weakness in extending, abducting, and adducting the hand at the wrist may occur because of partial loss of action of the chief extensors of the hand

132

(extensor carpi radialis longus and brevis, and extensor carpi ulnaris), two of the chief abductors of the hand (extensor carpi radialis longus and brevis), and one of the chief adductors of the hand (extensor carpi ulnaris). Weakness in supinating the forearm may occur because of partial loss of action of one of the two supinators of the forearm (supinator). Weakness in flexing the hand will not occur because none of the flexors of the hand are innervated by either the radial nerve or its branches.

Wrist drop occurs from injuries to the radial nerve which cause significant loss of action of the chief extensors of the hand. In wrist drop, the hand cannot be extended or can be only weakly extended at the wrist. Brachioradialis can flex the forearm and stabilize it in the midprone position. It does not exert any action across the wrist joint.

Items 273-276

In Items 273-276, match each set of symptoms in the items with the nerve listed below whose entrapment in the elbow or upper forearm would **MOST** likely lead to the set of symptoms. Answers may be used once, more than once, or not at all.

(A)	Median nerve
(B)	Ulnar nerve
(C)	Musculocutaneous nerve
(D)	Radial nerve
(E)	Anterior interosseous nerve
(F)	Posterior interosseous nerve

273.   In which nerve on the right could entrapment lead to decreased sensation to touch on the palmar surfaces of the thumb and index finger?

274.   In which nerve on the right could entrapment lead to weakened flexion of the thumb at its interphalangeal joint but **NO** cutaneous sensory deficits?

275.   In which nerve on the right could entrapment lead to decreased sensation to touch on the palmar surface of the little finger?

276.   In which nerve on the right could entrapment lead to weakened extension of the fingers but **NO** cutaneous sensory deficits?

ANSWERS AND TUTORIAL ON ITEMS 273-276

The answers are: **273-A; 274-E; 275-B; 276-F**. Item 273: Branches of the **median nerve** in the hand and lower forearm innervate the palmar surfaces of the thumb, index finger, middle finger, and lateral half of the ring finger and the lateral two-thirds of the palm (**Figure 3.18A**, shown in black). It is the only nerve whose entrapment in the elbow or upper forearm could lead to decreased sensation to touch on the palmar surfaces of the thumb and index finger. The median nerve can become entrapped where it passes between the humeral and ulnar heads of pronator teres in the upper forearm. This entrapment can lead to the **pronator teres syndrome** which is characterized by sensory deficits in one or more of the cutaneous areas of the hand that are innervated by branches of the median nerve.

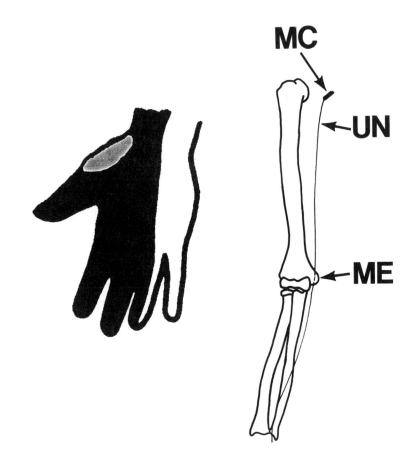

Figure 3.18A   **Figure 3.18B**

Item 274: The **anterior interosseus nerve** can become entrapped near its origin from the median nerve in the upper forearm leading to **anterior interosseous nerve syndrome**. The anterior interosseous nerve innervates flexor pollicis longus, the lateral half of flexor digitorum profundus, and pronator quadratus. Consequently, entrapment of the anterior interosseous nerve can lead to weakened flexion of the thumb at its interphalangeal joint or of the index and middle fingers at their distal interphalangeal joints. It can also lead to weakened pronation of the

134

forearm, but does not produce any cutaneous sensory deficits because the nerve does have any such branches.

Item 275: Branches of the **ulnar nerve** innervate the palmar surfaces of the little finger and medial half of the ring finger and the medial third of the palm (**Figure 3.18B**) and thus is the only nerve whose entrapment in the elbow or upper forearm could lead to decreased (**Figure 3.18A**) sensation to touch on the palmar surface of the little finger. As the ulnar nerve (UN) extends across the elbow region, it passes directly posterior to the medial epicondyle (ME) of the humerus in a groove that is converted into a passageway called the cubital tunnel by a ligament that extends from the medial epicondyle to the olecranon process of the ulna (**Figure 3.18B**). The ulnar nerve is subject to entrapment along its course through the cubital tunnel leading to **cubital tunnel syndrome** which is characterized by sensory deficits in the cutaneous areas of the hand that are innervated by branches of the ulnar nerve.

Item 276: Before discussing the entrapment syndromes involving the radial and posterior interosseous nerves, let us review the muscles and cutaneous areas innervated by the radial nerve and its branches. In the arm, the **radial nerve** innervates triceps brachii, brachioradialis, and extensor carpi radialis longus. In the arm, the radial nerve also gives rise to three cutaneous branches: the posterior cutaneous nerve of the arm (which innervates skin on the posterior surface of the arm), the lower lateral cutaneous nerve of the arm (which innervates the skin of the lower lateral aspect of the arm), and the posterior cutaneous nerve of the forearm (which innervates skin on the posterior surface of the forearm).

The radial nerve extends into the forearm by passing through the lateral side of the cubital fossa. At this level in the upper limb, the radial nerve divides into superficial radial and deep radial nerves. The superficial radial nerve is a cutaneous branch that innervates, in particular, the lateral aspect of the dorsum of the hand. The **deep radial nerve** innervates two posterior forearm muscles: extensor carpi radialis brevis and supinator.

Upon passing through supinator, the deep radial nerve becomes the posterior interosseous nerve which innervates extensor carpi ulnaris, abductor pollicis longus, extensor pollicis brevis, extensor pollicis longus, extensor indicis, extensor digitorum, and extensor digiti minimi. The posterior interosseous nerve does not have any cutaneous sensory branches.

The **radial** and **posterior interosseous nerves** are subject to entrapment near the elbow which can lead to sensory deficits in the skin areas supplied by the superficial radial nerve and to weakness in the muscles supplied by the deep radial and posterior interosseous nerves. Entrapment of the posterior interosseous nerve can lead to weakness of the muscles it innervates but no cutaneous sensory deficits. Observe that entrapment of either the radial nerve or the posterior interosseous nerve could lead to weakness in extension of the fingers. Entrapment of the radial nerve, however, could also lead to sensory deficits on the lateral aspect of the dorsum of the hand.

Entrapment of the musculocutaneous nerve: As the musculocutaneous nerve descends through the arm, it first gives rise to branches that innervate the anterior arm muscles (coracobrachialis, biceps brachii, and brachialis) and then becomes a wholly sensory nerve called the **lateral cutaneous nerve of the forearm**. It is subject to entrapment deep to the bicipital aponeurosis in the elbow which can lead to discomfort over the lateral aspect of the forearm. At this site, the musculocutaneous nerve has become the lateral cutaneous nerve of the forearm, and thus transmits only cutaneous sensory fibers from the lateral aspect of the forearm.

Choose the **BEST** response.

277.   A young man suffers a transverse cut across the anterior surface of the wrist that severs the major nerve which lies superficial to the flexor retinaculum. Which of the following actions will be **LOST** as a result of the severing of this major nerve?

    (A)   extending the fingers at their interphalangeal joints
    (B)   spreading apart the fingers (abducting the fingers)
    (C)   flexing the fingers at their interphalangeal joints
    (D)   abducting the hand at the wrist
    (E)   adducting the hand at the wrist

278.   An elderly women suffers partial paralysis of certain hand muscles because of compression of the major nerve which passes through the carpal tunnel in the wrist. Which of the following actions can be **WEAKENED** by injury to this major nerve?

    (A)   touching the base of the little finger with the tip of the thumb
    (B)   flexing the thumb at its interphalangeal joint
    (C)   adducting the thumb
    (D)   flexing the hand at the wrist
    (E)   abducting the hand at the wrist

ANSWERS AND TUTORIAL ON ITEMS 277-278

The answers are: **277-B; 278-A**. The median and ulnar nerves are the major nerves that extend across the wrist into the hand. Upon entering the hand, the nerves give rise to motor branches that innervate the hand muscles and cutaneous sensory branches that innervate the skin of the thumb and fingers.

Item 277 highlights one of the major motor deficits that may occur from injury to the **ulnar nerve** at any site along its course through the upper limb, namely, weakness or inability to abduct and adduct the fingers.

The ulnar nerve (UN) and ulnar artery (UA) cross the wrist by extending anterior to the flexor retinaculum (**Figure 3.19**). Upon entering the hand, the ulnar nerve divides into a superficial branch and a deep branch. The deep branch of the ulnar nerve innervates 13 hand muscles. They are

        1)   all 3 palmar interossei,
        2)   all 4 dorsal interossei,

3)   the 3rd and 4th lumbricals,
4)   the 3 muscles of the hypothenar eminence (abductor digiti minimi, flexor digiti minimi, and opponens digiti minimi)
5)   and adductor pollicis.

The dorsal interossei and abductor digiti minimi are the muscles which abduct the fingers at the metacarpophalangeal joints.

An injury to the ulnar nerve may lead to a **claw hand** primarily because of the paralysis of the 3rd and 4th lumbricals. The mechanism is as follows: The lumbricals act chiefly as flexors of the fingers at their metacarpophalangeal (MP) joints. If the 3rd and 4th lumbricals become paralyzed, they no longer resist the extensor action that extensor digitorum exerts at the MP joints of the two fingers and that extensor digiti minimi exerts at the MP joint of the little finger. The result is that the two fingers become hyperextended at their MP joints. Hyperextension at the MP joints stretches the flexor digitorum superficialis and profundus tendons that cross the anterior aspect of these joints, and thus the two fingers also become partially flexed at their interphalangeal (IP) joints. The ring and little fingers are thus forced into a claw configuration in which each finger is hyperextended at its MP joint and partially flexed at its IP joints.

Item 278 highlights one of the major motor deficits that may occur from injury to the **median nerve** at any site along its course through the upper limb, namely, weakness or inability to bring the tip of the thumb into contact with the fingers.

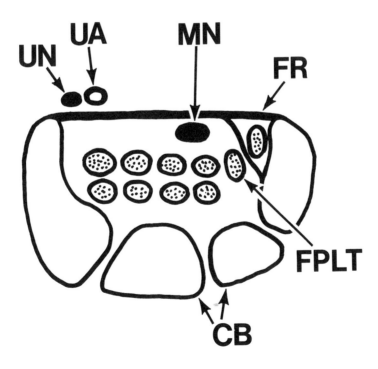

Figure 3.19

137

The median nerve (MN) crosses the wrist by extending through the **carpal tunnel (Figure 3.19)**, an osseofascial corridor in the wrist bordered anteriorly by the flexor retinaculum (FR) and posteriorly by the carpal bones (CB) (**Figure 3.19**). The major structures that pass through it are the median nerve, the 4 tendons of flexor digitorum superficialis, the 4 tendons of flexor digitorum profundus, and the tendon of flexor pollicis longus (FPLT).

Upon entering the hand, the median nerve innervates 5 hand muscles. They are the 3 muscles of the thenar eminence (abductor pollicis brevis, flexor pollicis brevis, and opponens pollicis), and the 1st and 2nd lumbricals. Opponens pollicis is the muscle which (in concert with other muscles) permits a person to touch the base of the little finger with the tip of the thumb.

Carpal tunnel syndrome involves sensory and/or motor deficits that occur as a consequence of compression on the median nerve as it passes through the carpal tunnel. The major sensory deficits occur on the palmar aspects of the thumb, index finger, and middle finger. The major motor deficits are weakness and difficulty in the use of the thumb to grasp and hold objects.

An injury that destroys all the motor nerve fibers in the median nerve leads to **ape hand**, primarily because of the paralysis of the muscles of the thenar eminence. The mechanism is as follows: The muscles of the thenar eminence play a major role in abducting, flexing, and medially rotating the thumb at its carpometacarpal joint. These actions move the thumb anterior to the palm of the hand and help bring the tip of the thumb into contact with the fingers. If the muscles of the thenar eminence are paralyzed, they no longer resist the adductor action of adductor pollicis and the tendency of abductor pollicis longus and extensor pollicis longus to laterally rotate the thumb at its carpometacarpal joint. The result is that the thumb is forced into a position immediately lateral to the palm of the hand.

Items 279-284

An 8-year-old girl's right hand is clawed by a cat. Later there is evidence of lymphatic dissemination of a hand infection.

Choose the **BEST** response.

279. If superficial tissues on the medial aspect of the palm of the girl's hand are infected, which of the following groups of lymph nodes will **COMMONLY** be the first to react to lymphatic dissemination of the infection?

   (A)   anterior axillary
   (B)   lateral axillary
   (C)   deltopectoral (infraclavicular) axillary
   (D)   central axillary
   (E)   supratrochlear

280. Which group of lymph nodes will **COMMONLY** be the first to react to lymphatic dissemination of an infection of deep tissues in the hand?

    (A)   anterior axillary
    (B)   lateral axillary
    (C)   deltopectoral (infraclavicular) axillary
    (D)   central axillary
    (E)   supratrochlear

281. Superficial lymph nodes which are mounting an immunological response to infectious agents generally exhibit all of the following characteristics **EXCEPT**:

    (A)   enlarged
    (B)   irregularly shaped
    (C)   tender
    (D)   relatively mobile
    (E)   firm consistency

282. Which group of axillary lymph nodes is clustered about the region where the cephalic vein pierces deep fascia to extend toward its union with the axillary vein?

    (A)   anterior
    (B)   posterior
    (C)   lateral
    (D)   central
    (E)   deltopectoral (infraclavicular)

283. Which group of axillary lymph nodes is palpable against the anterior aspect of the posterior axillary fold?

    (A)   anterior
    (B)   posterior
    (C)   lateral
    (D)   central
    (E)   deltopectoral (infraclavicular)

284. Which group of axillary lymph nodes is the **FIRST** to receive lymph drained from the lateral half of the mammary gland?

    (A)   anterior
    (B)   posterior
    (C)   lateral
    (D)   central
    (E)   deltopectoral (infraclavicular)

The answers are: **279-E; 280-B; 281-B; 282-E; 283-B; 284-A**. Lymph nodes mounting an immunological response are enlarged but regularly shaped, tender, relatively mobile, and firm. Normal superficial lymph nodes are frequently small and therefore difficult to palpate, non-tender, relatively mobile, and soft. There are 7 groups of **lymph nodes** located in the upper limb. These lymph nodes collectively drain all the tissues of the upper limb, the ipsilateral superficial tissues of the chest wall, the superficial tissues of the anterior abdominal wall down to the level of the umbilicus, and the ipsilateral posterior abdominal wall down to the upper margin of the buttock.

1) The **supratrochlear lymph nodes** are the most distal lymph nodes in the upper limb. They can be palpated along the medial side of the basilic vein immediately superior to the medial epicondyle of the humerus. They drain superficial tissues of the medial aspect of the hand and forearm. All of the other 6 groups of upper limb lymph nodes are located in the axilla.

2) The **lateral group** of axillary lymph nodes is the most lateral group of lymph nodes in the axilla. They can be palpated along the medial side of the head of the humerus. They drain the deep tissues of the hand, forearm, and arm; the superficial tissues of the medial aspect of the hand, forearm, arm; and the supratrochlear nodes.

3) The **anterior** (pectoral) **group** of axillary nodes can be palpated against the posterior aspect of the anterior axillary fold. They drain the superficial tissues of the anterior aspect of the trunk, down to the level of the umbilicus and are typically involved in lymphatic dissemination of malignant cells from tumors that arise in the lateral half of the mammary gland.

4) The **posterior** (subscapular) **group** of axillary nodes can be palpated against the anterior aspect of the posterior axillary fold. They drain the superficial tissues of the posterior aspect of the trunk, down to the level of the iliac crest.

5) The **central group** of axillary nodes can be palpated in the center of the axilla against the chest wall. They drain the lateral, anterior, and posterior groups of axillary nodes.

6) The **deltopectoral group** of axillary nodes can be palpated directly below the midregion of the clavicle, which is where the cephalic vein pierces deep fascia to extend toward its union with the axillary vein. They drain the superficial tissues of the lateral aspect of the hand, forearm, and arm.

7) The **apical group** of axillary nodes lies along the axillary vein, immediately lateral to the first rib. They drain all the other axillary nodes.

In the following items, match each carpal bone with its image in **Figure 3.20**.

285. Scaphoid

286. Capitate

287. Lunate

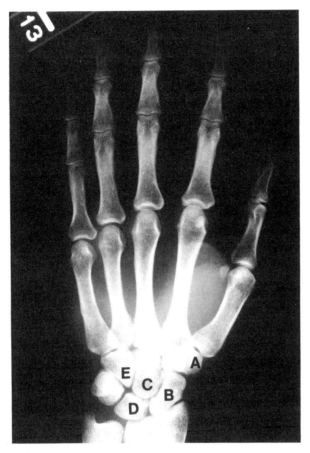

Figure 3.20

ANSWERS AND TUTORIAL ON ITEMS 285-287

The answers are: **285-B; 286-C; 287-D. Figure 3.20** is a labeled PA radiograph of the hand. The carpal bone labeled A is the **trapezium**, and the bone labeled E is the **hamate**.

The **scaphoid** (B) is the most commonly fractured carpal bone, and the **lunate** (D) is the most commonly dislocated carpal bone. The **capitate** (C) is the largest carpal bone. Note that the central axes of the third metacarpal and capitate are parallel and project proximally between the scaphoid and lunate.

The trapezium, scaphoid, and styloid process of the radius form the bony floor of the **anatomical snuffbox** of the wrist. In the wrist joint, the scaphoid, lunate, and **triquetrum** articulate with the distal end of the radius and the triangular disk of fibrocartilage.

Items 288-296

The following items pertain to the anatomy of the hip and inguinal regions of the lower limb.

Choose the **BEST** response.

288. All of the following statements concerning the limits of passive movement at the hip joint in a normal young adult are correct **EXCEPT**:

    (A)   The thigh can be externally rotated approximately 45°.
    (B)   The thigh can be internally rotated approximately 40°.
    (C)   If the leg is flexed 90° at the knee, the thigh can be passively flexed approximately 120°.
    (D)   If the leg is fully extended (is at 0° flexion at the knee), the thigh can be passively flexed approximately 45°.
    (E)   The thigh can be abducted approximately 45°.

289. Which movement of the thigh at the hip joint can be weakened by impingement of the first lumbar spinal nerve?

    (A)   flexion
    (B)   extension
    (C)   abduction
    (D)   adduction
    (E)   external rotation

290. A patient has a one lower limb that appears shorter than the other because of reflexive contraction of medial thigh muscles in the shorter limb. One can assess whether the lower limbs actually differ in length by measuring the length from the _____ to the medial malleolus.

    (A)   iliac tubercle
    (B)   pubic tubercle
    (C)   pubis symphysis
    (D)   anterior superior iliac spine
    (E)   anterior inferior iliac spine

291. Hip joint pain can be referred to all of the following regions **EXCEPT**:

    (A)   umbilicus
    (B)   lower back
    (C)   groin
    (D)   thigh
    (E)   knee

292. An enlarged lymph node in the horizontal group of superficial inguinal nodes in a male could be the result of a disease in all of the following regions **EXCEPT**:

(A) anterior abdominal wall inferior to the umbilicus
(B) penis
(C) testis
(D) buttock
(E) anal canal

293. An enlarged lymph node in the vertical group of superficial inguinal nodes in a female could be the result of a disease in all of the following regions **EXCEPT**:

(A) anterior surface of the thigh
(B) posterior surface of the thigh
(C) medial surface of the leg
(D) superficial tissues on the lateral side of the foot
(E) superficial tissues on the medial side of the foot

294. A patient is given an inappropriate intramuscular injection in the buttock midway between the ischial tuberosity and greater trochanter of the femur which elicits an inflammatory reaction in a nerve deep to the injection site and produces pain that radiates from the buttock down the posterolateral aspect of the thigh. Which nerve is inflamed?

(A) lateral femoral cutaneous nerve
(B) femoral nerve
(C) sciatic nerve
(D) obturator nerve
(E) pudendal nerve

295. The femoral vein can be catheterized in the upper thigh. At the site where the needle is typically inserted into the femoral vein, all of the following relationships are correct **EXCEPT**:

(A) The femoral vein lies deep to the fascia lata of the thigh.
(B) The femoral vein lies anterior to a muscle that intervenes between the vein and the capsule of the hip joint.
(C) The femoral vein lies directly medial to the femoral artery.
(D) The femoral vein lies directly lateral to the femoral canal.
(E) The femoral vein lies (in an adult) about two finger breadths lateral to the femoral nerve.

296. All of the following disorders can produce a positive Trendelenburg's sign **EXCEPT**:

(A) paralysis of gluteus medius and gluteus minimus
(B) ischial bursitis
(C) an abnormal angle of inclination between the neck and shaft of the femur
(D) dislocation of the hip joint
(E) osteoarthritis of the hip joint

ANSWERS AND TUTORIAL ON ITEMS 288-296

The answers are: **288-D; 289-A; 290-D; 291-A; 292-C; 293-D; 294-C; 295-E; 296-B**. Item 288: If the leg is fully extended at the knee, the thigh can be passively flexed approximately 90° before tension in the hamstring muscles (semitendinosus, semimembranosus, and the long head of biceps femoris) becomes painful and limits further flexion.

Item 289: The spinal nerves **L1** and **L2** provide most of the innervation for the major flexors of the thigh: iliacus and psoas major. Iliacus is innervated primarily by L2 nerve fibers, and psoas major is innervated primarily by L1 and L2 nerve fibers. Some physicians assess flexion of the thigh against resistance as a test of L1 innervation of psoas major.

L5, S1, and **S2** provide most of the innervation for the major extensors of the thigh: gluteus maximus and the hamstrings. Gluteus maximus is innervated primarily by S1 and S2 fibers, semitendinosus and semimembranosus are innervated primarily by L5 and S1 fibers, and the long head of biceps femoris is innervated primarily by S1 fibers.

L5 fibers provide most of the innervation for both of the major abductors of the thigh: gluteus medius and gluteus minimus.

L2, L3, and **L4** provide most of the innervation for the major adductors of the thigh: adductor magnus, adductor brevis, adductor longus, and gracilis. Adductor magnus is innervated primarily by L3 and L4 fibers, adductor brevis and adductor longus are innervated primarily by L3 fibers, and gracilis is innervated primarily by L2 fibers.

S1 fibers provide most of the innervation for the external rotators of the thigh: piriformis, superior gemellus, obturator internus, inferior gemellus, and quadratus femoris.

Item 290: **Pelvic obliquity** (one side of the pelvis being lower than the other side) and reflexive contraction of the major adductors of the thigh are conditions which functionally foreshorten a lower limb. A patient suffering from either condition thus may appear to have lower limbs of unequal length. The true, anatomical lengths of the lower limbs can be compared by measuring the length of each limb from the anterior superior iliac spine to the medial malleolus.

Item 291: Disease or injury of an internal structure may at times lead to **referred pain** in skin areas whose sensory innervation arises from the same spinal cord segments that provide sensory innervation for the internal structure. The **hip joint** is innervated by branches of the femoral nerve, obturator nerve, nerve to quadratus femoris, and superior gluteal nerve. The femoral and obturator nerves transmit sensory fibers that enter the spinal cord at the L2, L3, and

L4 levels, and the nerve to quadratus femoris and the superior gluteal nerve transmit sensory fibers that enter the spinal cord at the L5 and S1 levels. Disease or injury of the hip joint may thus refer pain to parts of the L2, L3, L4, L5, and S1 **dermatomes**.

Disease or injury of the hip joint refers pain most commonly to the groin; other regions of referred pain include the lower back, thigh, knee, and even the ankle. The skin overlying these regions represents parts of the L2, L3, L4, L5, or S1 dermatomes. The skin around the umbilicus is part of the T10 dermatome.

Items 292 and 293: There are 4 groups of **lymph nodes** located in the lower limb. These lymph nodes collectively drain all the tissues of the lower limb, the superficial tissues of the anterior abdominal wall (up to the level of the umbilicus) and buttock on the ipsilateral (same) side of the body, the external genitalia (but NOT the testis in a male), the urethra, and the lower half of the anal canal.

1) The **popliteal nodes** are the most distal lymph nodes in the lower limb and can be palpated in the popliteal fossa when the leg is flexed about 90° at the knee. They drain the deep tissues of the leg and foot and the superficial tissues on the lateral side of the foot and the posterolateral aspect of the leg.

2) The **vertical group of superficial inguinal nodes** can be palpated in the superficial fascia of the upper, anterior aspect of the thigh alongside the terminal segment of the great saphenous vein. They drain all the superficial tissues of the lower limb except for those on the lateral side of the foot and the posterolateral aspect of the leg.

3) The **horizontal group of superficial inguinal nodes** can be palpated in the superficial fascia of the upper, anterior aspect of the thigh just below the inguinal ligament. They drain the superficial tissues of the anterior abdominal wall (up to the level of the umbilicus) and buttock, the external genitalia (except for the testis in a male), the urethra, and the lower half of the anal canal.

4) The **deep group of inguinal nodes** lies alongside the terminal segment of the femoral vein in the front of the thigh. They drain lymph from the popliteal nodes, the deep tissues of the thigh, and some of the superficial inguinal nodes. The lymph nodes that drain the testis lie in the retroperitoneal space of the abdomen, near the site where the testicular artery arises from the abdominal aorta.

Item 294: One of the most serious complications of intramuscular injections in the buttock is inflammation of the **sciatic nerve**. Injections should be made in the upper lateral quadrant of the buttock, which is the quadrant furthest from the course of the sciatic nerve through the buttock. The sciatic nerve follows a downward curving course through the lower medial quadrant of the buttock and then enters the back of the thigh at a point midway between the greater trochanter of the femur and the ischial tuberosity.

Item 295: The **femoral vein** can be catheterized under emergency conditions to administer large volumes of fluid quickly. The femoral vein is accessed in the upper front of the thigh, where the vein lies directly medial to the femoral artery. If the pulsations of the femoral artery can be palpated, the needle is inserted (in an adult) at a site about 2 cm medial to the femoral pulse and 3 to 4 cm below the inguinal ligament. If the femoral pulse cannot be palpated, it is useful to remember that the femoral artery enters the thigh beneath the inguinal ligament at the midpoint between the anterior superior iliac spine and pubic symphysis.

In the front of the thigh, the femoral vein lies directly lateral to the femoral canal, which is the space that harbors the deep inguinal lymph nodes. The femoral nerve lies lateral to the femoral artery, entering the thigh beneath the inguinal ligament at the midpoint between the anterior superior iliac spine and pubic tubercle. Psoas major is the muscle that intervenes between the femoral vein and the capsule of the hip joint.

Item 296: When a person attempts to stand (or support the body) on one lower limb only, gluteus medius and minimus (the chief abductors of the thigh) on the side of the supporting lower limb tense to elevate the contralateral side of the pelvis. This tilting of the pelvis balances the body over the supporting lower limb. An inability to tilt the pelvis in this fashion is called **Trendelenburg's sign**. Any disorder which limits the capacity of gluteus medius and minimus to support and steady the body when standing on the ipsilateral lower limb or produces pain in the hip joint when it bears the weight of the upper body may produce Trendelenburg's sign. Ischial bursitis is inflammation of the ischial bursa, which lies just superficial to the ischial tuberosity.

Items 297-299

The parents of a 6-year-old boy, in good health until recently, now report that he has started walking with a limp. His temperature is 98.5° F. He walks with a limp because of right hip pain. The hip pain is aggravated by weight-bearing and relieved by rest. Trendelenburg's sign is observed when the boy is asked to stand on the right lower limb only. Radiographs of the hip joints show periarticular soft tissue swelling about the right hip joint. A bone scan reveals diminished activity in the anterolateral aspect of the right capital femoral epiphysis.

297. The **MOST** likely diagnosis is

    (A) transient synovitis of the hip joint
    (B) septic arthritis of the hip joint
    (C) Legg-Calvé-Perthes disease
    (D) a slipped capital femoral epiphysis
    (E) epiphyseal dysplasia

298. The **CHIEF** source of blood supply to this boy's capital femoral epiphysis are

    (A) arteries in the ligament to the head of the femur
    (B) medullary arteries of the metaphysis
    (C) arteries derived from the medial and lateral circumflex femoral arteries
    (D) arteries derived from the superior gluteal artery
    (E) arteries derived from the inferior gluteal artery

146

299. Which of the following positions of the right thigh will minimize this boy's lower limb pain?

   (A) completely extended and slightly internally rotated
   (B) completely extended and neutrally rotated
   (C) completely extended and slightly internally rotated
   (D) flexed 90° and slightly externally rotated
   (E) flexed 90° and slightly internally rotated

ANSWERS AND TUTORIAL ON ITEMS 297-299

The answers are: **297-C; 298-C; 299-D**. **Legg-Calvé-Perthes disease** is a self-limiting hip disorder of children involving vascular compromise of the capital femoral epiphysis. Diminished vascularization in the anterolateral aspect of the capital femoral epiphysis is characteristic of the pattern of ischemic necrosis which occurs in Legg-Calvé-Perthes disease. The radiographic evidence of periarticular soft tissue swelling suggests that the patient is also suffering from inflammation of the synovial membrane and effusion of the hip joint.

The etiology of Legg-Calvé-Perthes disease is unknown. The anatomical basis of the disorder is believed to be related to the developmental changes in the blood supply to the hip during childhood. Branches of the **medial** and **lateral circumflex femoral arteries** form an extracapsular vascular ring around the base of the neck of the femur. Branches of the extracapsular vascular ring called the **retinacular arteries** ascend along the neck of the femur to penetrate the capsule of the hip joint and give rise within the joint to branches that supply the upper end of the femur. The retinacular arteries and their branches are believed to be the chief source of blood supply to the head of the femur at all ages. At birth, the cartilaginous femoral head is also supplied by arteries entering the head from the shaft of the femur. Establishment of the epiphyseal plate between the capital epiphysis and the metaphysis by about 4 years of age abolishes all blood supply from the metaphysis. This arrangement persists until about 9 years of age, at which time the arteries in the ligament to the head of the femur begin to become increasingly prominent in supplying the head of the femur. **Medullary arteries of the metaphysis** begin to supply the femoral head upon epiphyseal fusion in late adolescence or early adulthood. The childhood period from 4 to 9 years of age, when the retinacular arteries are the sole significant source of blood supply to the capital epiphysis, spans the years of the highest incidence of Legg-Calvé-Perthes disease.

Much of the patient's right hip pain is emanating from tension in the joint's inflamed synovial membrane which is minimized when the thigh is flexed 90° and slightly externally rotated. Accordingly, patients with a painful hip effusion are generally most comfortable when seated with the painful thigh slightly externally rotated. Active and passive attempts at internal rotation or abduction of the thigh commonly exacerbate the lower limb pain of patients with Legg-Calvé-Perthes disease.

Items 300-304

The following items pertain to the anatomy of the knee.

Choose the **BEST** response.

300.   All of the following statements concerning the limits of passive movement at the knee joint of a normal young adult are correct **EXCEPT**:

(A)   The leg can be flexed approximately 130°.
(B)   The leg can be hyperextended 10 to 15°.
(C)   If the leg is flexed 90°, it can be internally rotated approximately 30°.
(D)   If the leg is flexed 90°, it can be externally rotated approximately 40°.
(E)   If the leg is fully extended, it can be internally or externally rotated approximately 45°.

301.   The quadriceps femoris deep tendon reflex involves sensory and motor nerve fibers in spinal nerves

(A)   L1, L2 and L3
(B)   L2, L3 and L4
(C)   L3, L4 and L5
(D)   L4, L5 and S1
(E)   L5, S1 and S2

302.   Strengthening which muscle would relieve recurrent patellar subluxation due to muscular disuse atrophy?

(A)   semitendinosus
(B)   gracilis
(C)   vastus medialis
(D)   vastus lateralis
(E)   sartorius

303.   An effusion of the synovial cavity of the knee joint may result in all of the following **EXCEPT**:

(A)   A swelling of the soft tissues directly anterior to the patella.
(B)   A swelling along the upper margin of the patella.
(C)   Swellings along the medial or lateral sides of the patella.
(D)   Swellings along the medial or lateral sides of the patellar ligament.
(E)   Displacement of the patella anterior from the intercondylar area of the femur.

148

304. All of the following conditions can produce a swelling in the popliteal fossa. Which condition can be distinguished from all the others by gentle palpation of the swelling for a period of 10 to 15 seconds?

(A)   arterial aneurysm
(B)   venous thrombus
(C)   inflamed bursa
(D)   inflamed lymph node
(E)   Baker's cyst

ANSWERS AND TUTORIAL ON ITEMS 300-304

The answers are: **300-E; 301-B; 302-C; 303-A; 304-A**. Item 300: When the **knee joint** is fully extended it is most stable because the femoral condyles are in maximal contact with the meniscotibial surfaces because the anterior and posterior cruciate ligaments, the medial and lateral collateral ligaments and the oblique popliteal ligament are all in part twisted and tightly stretched across the knee. The leg is externally rotated to the maximum extent within the knee joint and thus no internal or external rotation of the leg is possible. Assessment of passive internal and external rotation of the leg at the knee is conducted with the leg flexed 90°.

Items 301 and 302: The 4 muscles that form the **quadriceps femoris** (rectus femoris, vastus medialis, vastus intermedius and vastus lateralis) share a common tendon of insertion that partially envelops the patella before inserting onto the tibial tuberosity. Quadriceps femoris is the sole extensor of the leg and is innervated by the femoral nerve (L2, L3 and L4).

When the quadriceps femoris muscles extend the leg at the knee, the medially-directed tug exerted by vastus medialis counterbalances the laterally-directed tug exerted by vastus intermedius and lateralis. When disease or injury of the knee leads to disuse atrophy of muscles that act across the knee joint, vastus medialis is the first of the quadriceps femoris muscles to atrophy and the last to recover. The diminishment of the medially-directed tug on the patella by vastus medialis can lead, in turn, to recurrent, lateral subluxation of the patella during leg extension.

Item 303: When **fluid accumulates** in the synovial cavity of the knee joint, the normal hollowed contours around the patella and along the sides of the patellar ligament may swell and the patella may be displaced anteriorly. The contours surrounding the upper margin of the patella may swell because of expansion of the underlying suprapatellar bursa. The suprapatellar bursa is an extension of the knee joint's synovial cavity. The bursa lies deep to the quadriceps femoris tendon and extends for about 5-7 cm above the upper border of the patella. The hollowed contours along the sides of the patellar ligament may swell because the knee joint's synovial membrane lining extends inferiorly along both sides of the infrapatellar fat pad, which lies deep to the patellar ligament. The patella may be displaced anteriorly because the patella and the portion of the quadriceps femoris tendon in which it is embedded form the anterior aspect of the knee joint. The subcutaneous tissues that overlie the patella lie superficial to the knee joint and thus do not swell when the knee joint has an effusion. The prepatellar bursa lies in the subcutaneous tissues that overlie the patella, but the prepatellar bursa does not communicate with the knee joint's synovial cavity.

Item 304: The most common conditions which can produce a **swelling in the popliteal fossa** are an aneurysm of the popliteal artery, a thrombus in the popliteal vein, an inflamed bursa, an inflamed lymph node (for a discussion of popliteal lymph nodes, see the tutorial for Items 292 and 293), and a **Baker's cyst**. A Baker's cyst is a fluid-filled herniation of the synovial membrane lining the posterior aspect of the knee joint. The only swelling that pulses is an **aneurysm of the popliteal artery**.

Figure 3.21 shows T1-weighted magnetic resonance images (MRIs) of coronal (A) and sagittal (B) sections of the **NORMAL** knee. A patient received a strong blow to the lateral side of her knee when it was weight-bearing and partially flexed. Match the labeled structure in the MRIs below with the physical findings described in the clinical scenarios in the items.

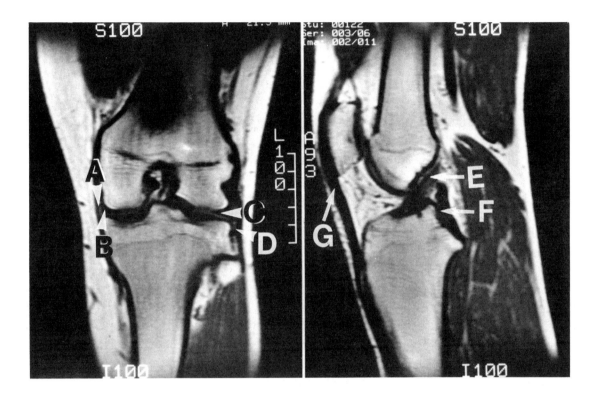

Figure 3.21

305.   Application of a valgus stress with the knee flexed 30° produces abnormal medial widening of the knee joint, suggesting a tear in _____.

306.   With the knee flexed 30°, when the leg is pulled forward, there is a "mushy" or "soft" feel at the end point of anterior movement, suggesting a tear in _____.

ANSWERS AND TUTORIAL ON ITEMS 305-306

The answers are: **305-A; 306-E**. The labeled structures in **Figures 3.21A** and **3.21B** are:

A - medial collateral ligament
B - medial meniscus
C - lateral meniscus
D - lateral collateral ligament
E - anterior cruciate ligament
F - posterior cruciate ligament
G - patellar ligament

The **medial collateral ligament** (A) of the knee acts to keep the medial femoral and medial tibial condyles in close contact with each other. It is susceptible to injury from blows to the lateral side of the knee when the knee is weight-bearing and partially flexed because such blows force apart the medial femoral and tibial condyles and thus put a severe strain upon the medial collateral ligament. The integrity of the medial collateral ligament is tested by applying a **valgus stress** with the knee flexed 30° (medially-directed force at the knee simultaneously with a laterally-directed force at the ankle). When the knee is flexed 30°, the medial and lateral collateral ligaments are the most effective ligamentous supports, respectively, of medial and lateral stability of the knee. If a valgus stress produces an abnormal widening of the joint space in the medial aspect of the knee, then it is likely that the medial collateral ligament is significantly torn.

The **anterior cruciate ligament** (E) of the knee is an intracapsular ligament that extends from the internal surface of the lateral femoral condyle to the anterior area of the tibial intercondylar surface. It is susceptible to injury from blows to the lateral side of the knee when the knee is weight-bearing and partially flexed. Such blows stretch the anterior cruciate ligament across the internal surface of the lateral femoral condyle. The integrity of the anterior cruciate ligament is tested by pulling the leg forward at the knee with the knee flexed 30°. A 'soft' or 'mushy' feel to the end point of the anterior movement of the leg suggests a significant tear of the anterior cruciate ligament.

The following items address the anatomy of the leg, ankle, and foot.

Choose the **BEST** response.

307.   The pair of muscles **CHIEFLY** responsible for inversion of the foot are

    (A)   tibialis anterior and tibialis posterior
    (B)   plantaris and quadratus plantae
    (C)   gastrocnemius and soleus
    (D)   peroneus longus and peroneus brevis
    (E)   extensor digitorum longus and flexor digitorum longus

308.   The pulsations of the posterior tibial artery can be palpated

    (A)   on the dorsum of the foot immediately lateral to the tendon of extensor hallucis longus
    (B)   posteroinferiorly to the lateral malleolus
    (C)   anterosuperiorly to the lateral malleolus
    (D)   posteroinferiorly to the medial malleolus
    (E)   anterosuperiorly to the medial malleolus

309.   The Achilles tendon stretch reflex involves sensory and motor fibers in spinal nerves

    (A)   L1 and L2
    (B)   L3 and L4
    (C)   S1 and S2
    (D)   S3 and S4
    (E)   S5

310.   **MOST** ankle sprains are produced by marked inversion of a supinated, plantarflexed foot. Which ligament is torn first by such a stress?

    (A)   deltoid ligament
    (B)   plantar calcaneonavicular ligament
    (C)   anterior talofibular ligament
    (D)   calcaneofibular ligament
    (E)   posterior talofibular ligament

ANSWERS AND TUTORIAL ON ITEMS 307-310

The answers are: **307-A; 308-D; 309-C; 310-C**. Item 307: Leg muscles are the prime movers of plantarflexion, dorsiflexion, inversion, and eversion of the foot. Gastrocnemius and soleus are the chief **plantarflexors** of the foot. Tibialis anterior, extensor hallucis longus, and extensor digitorum longus are the chief **dorsiflexors** of the foot. Peroneus longus and peroneus brevis are the chief evertors of the foot.

Item 308: The **posterior tibial artery** is the only artery whose pulsations can be reliably palpated at the ankle. The pulsations of dorsalis pedis can be generally palpated on the dorsum of the foot immediately lateral to the tendon of extensor hallucis longus.

Item 309: The chief muscles which insert onto the calcaneus via the Achilles tendon (gastrocnemius and soleus) are innervated by fibers of the tibial nerve derived principally from the **S1** and **S2** roots of the sacral plexus.

Item 310: Marked inversion of a supinated, plantarflexed foot stresses the three ligaments which form the **lateral collateral ligament** of the ankle joint. The stress typically tears the **anterior talofibular ligament** first, the calcaneofibular ligament second, and the posterior talofibular ligament third.

Items 311-314

A 29-year-old man sustains a severe compression injury to his left upper leg as a result of a fall from a motorcycle. Examination reveals a contusion surrounding the head and neck of the fibula.

Choose the **BEST** response.

311.   Which nerve is susceptible to direct injury by a severe compression force applied to the lateral aspect of the head and neck of the fibula?

   (A)   common peroneal nerve
   (B)   deep peroneal nerve
   (C)   superficial peroneal nerve
   (D)   tibial nerve
   (E)   saphenous nerve

312.   Injury to this nerve could result in weakness in all of the following movements **EXCEPT**:

   (A)   inversion of the foot
   (B)   eversion of the foot
   (C)   dorsiflexion of the foot
   (D)   flexion of the toes
   (E)   extension of the toes

154

313. Cutaneous branches of the deep peroneal nerve supply the

    (A)   medial side of the big toe
    (B)   adjacent sides of the big and 2nd toes
    (C)   adjacent sides of the 2nd and 3rd toes
    (D)   adjacent sides of the 3rd and 4th toes
    (E)   adjacent sides of the 4th and 5th toes

314. The dorsum of the foot is supplied by cutaneous branches of the

    (A)   superficial peroneal nerve
    (B)   deep peroneal nerve
    (C)   tibial nerve
    (D)   sural nerve
    (E)   saphenous nerve

ANSWERS AND TUTORIAL ON ITEMS 311-314

The answers are: **311-A; 312-D; 313-B; 314-A**. As the **common peroneal nerve** descends through the popliteal fossa, it parallels the medial border of biceps femoris's tendon of insertion. The common peroneal nerve (CPN) then curves inferolaterally around the head (H) and neck (N) of the fibula as it enters the leg (**Figure 3.22**). The common peroneal nerve ends in this vicinity by dividing into the **superficial** and **deep peroneal nerves**. The superficial peroneal nerve innervates peroneus longus and peroneus brevis, the major evertors of the foot. The deep peroneal nerve innervates all the dorsiflexors of the foot (tibialis anterior, extensor hallucis longus, extensor digitorum longus, and peroneus tertius) and extensor digitorum brevis. Tibialis anterior is one of the two major invertors of the foot. Extensor hallucis longus, extensor digitorum longus, and extensor digitorum brevis are the extensors of the toes. The superficial and deep peroneal nerves do not innervate any of the flexors of the toes. The flexors of the toes are all innervated by the tibial nerve or one of its two terminal branches, the medial and lateral plantar nerves. The adjacent sides of the big and 2nd toes are the only cutaneous areas of the foot supplied by cutaneous branches of the deep peroneal nerve. Cutaneous branches of the superficial peroneal nerve supply the dorsum of the foot. Cutaneous branches of the medial and lateral plantar nerves supply most of the sole of the foot.

    Foot drop occurs from injuries to the common peroneal nerve or deep peroneal nerve which cause significant loss of action of the chief dorsiflexors of the foot (tibialis anterior, extensor hallucis longus, and extensor digitorum longus). Foot drop is the condition in which the foot cannot be dorsiflexed or can be only weakly dorsiflexed at the ankle joint. This motor deficit significantly affects the walking gait because the foot cannot be maintained in a neutral position at the ankle as the foot is swung forward during the swing phase of the walking gait. Maintenance of a neutral position at the ankle causes the heel to be the first part of the foot to strike the ground following a step forward. With foot drop, the toes become the first part of the foot to strike the ground. Patients with foot drop compensate for the loss of dorsiflexion action by hyperflexing the thigh during the swing phase. This exaggerated movement plants the entire plantar surface of the foot on the ground following a step forward.

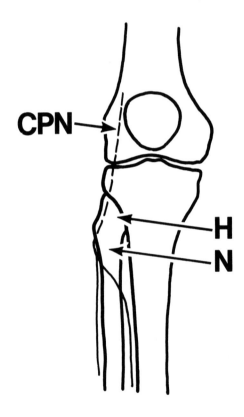

Figure 3.22

A 61-year-old man states that he likes to walk for exercise, but that recently he has pain in his right calf that appears after 10 minutes of walking. Resting for a few minutes alleviates the pain.

Choose the **BEST** response.

315. The **MOST** likely diagnosis for the patient's calf pain is

   (A)   an arterial aneurysm
   (B)   deep venous thrombosis
   (C)   incompetent valves in the deep veins
   (D)   peripheral atherosclerotic occlusive disease
   (E)   a tear of one of the heads of gastrocnemius

316. The patient suffers from a lesion involving the

   (A)   external iliac artery
   (B)   popliteal artery or femoral artery distal to the origin of profunda femoris
   (C)   profunda femoris
   (D)   anterior tibial artery
   (E)   posterior tibial artery

317. The cruciate anastomosis in the upper thigh is formed by the anastomosis of branches from all of the following arteries **EXCEPT**:

   (A)   medial circumflex femoral artery
   (B)   lateral circumflex femoral artery
   (C)   superior gluteal artery
   (D)   inferior gluteal artery
   (E)   first perforating branch of the profunda femoris

318. The peroneal artery in the leg is a branch of the

   (A)   femoral artery
   (B)   profunda femoris
   (C)   popliteal artery
   (D)   anterior tibial artery
   (E)   posterior tibial artery

The answers are: **315-D; 316-B; 317-C; 318-E. Peripheral atherosclerotic occlusive disease** is a condition in larger arteries of the extremities become occluded by plaques. The most common initial symptom of the disease in a lower limb is muscular pain or fatigue that occurs with exercise but abates with rest (intermittent claudication).

Occlusions in the **external iliac** (EI) **artery** diminish blood supply to almost all of the lower limb's muscles (**Figure 3.23**), and thus produce exertion-dependent pain extending distally from the buttock. Occlusions in the **femoral** (F) **artery** immediately proximal to the origin of profunda femoris (PF) (the deep femoral artery) diminish blood supply to the thigh and leg muscles, and thus produce exertion-dependent pain extending distally from the thigh. Occlusions in the **popliteal** (P) **artery** or femoral artery distal to the origin of profunda femoris produce exertion-dependent pain in the leg muscles. Progressive obstruction in the anterior or posterior **tibial arteries** does not diminish blood supply to the leg muscles, and thus does not produce intermittent claudication.

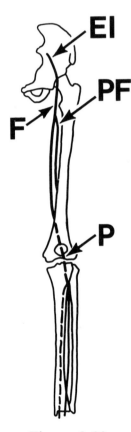

Figure 3.23

In the buttock and back of the thigh, the **superior** and **inferior gluteal** (SG and IG) **arteries**, the **medial** and **lateral circumflex femoral** (MCF and LCF) **arteries**, and the four perforating branches (PB) of the profunda femoris give rise to ascending and/or descending branches (**Figure 3.24**). The anastomoses among these ascending and descending branches form a vertical chain of arteries in the posterior compartment of the thigh which extends from branches of the internal iliac artery in the buttock to genicular branches of the **popliteal artery** in the knee region. The **cruciate anastomosis** is one of the major anastomoses in this vertical chain. Under emergency conditions, the femoral artery can be ligated at any point along its course through the anterior compartment of the thigh without risking total loss of blood supply to the lower limb distal to the site of ligation because the vertical chain of anastomosed arteries in the posterior compartment of the thigh provides collateral circulation to the knee, leg, and foot. The **peroneal artery** is a chief source of blood supply to the tissues of the lateral compartment of the leg. Peroneus longus and peroneus brevis are the only muscles here.

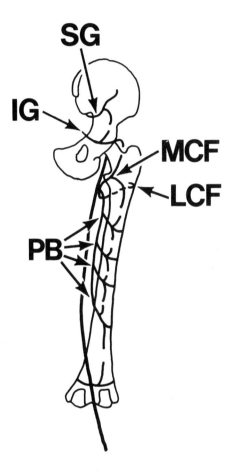

Figure 3.24

159

Items 319-322

Upon returning home after a 10-hour airline flight, a 55-year-old woman begins to experience pain the calf of the left leg that intensifies upon standing or walking. Examination reveals tachycardia (pulse of 90), fever (100.5° F) and cyanosis of the skin of the lower leg and foot.

Choose the **BEST** response.

319.	The **MOST** likely diagnosis for the patient's calf pain is

	(A)	an arterial aneurysm
	(B)	deep venous thrombosis
	(C)	incompetent valves in the deep veins
	(D)	Raynaud's disease
	(E)	a tear of one of the heads of gastrocnemius

320.	What is a possible complication of the patient's disorder?

	(A)	carotid embolism
	(B)	subclavian embolism
	(C)	pulmonary embolism
	(D)	superior mesenteric embolism
	(E)	femoral embolism

321.	Medium-sized and large veins of the lower limb may be palpated for tenderness in cases of suspected deep venous thrombosis. All of the following sites are appropriate for palpation of venous tenderness **EXCEPT**:

	(A)	region deep to the medial aspect of the Achilles tendon
	(B)	anterior region between the tibia and fibula in the lower leg
	(C)	calf region overlying the soleus muscle
	(D)	popliteal fossa
	(E)	region immediately lateral to the pulsations of the femoral artery along the superior border of the femoral triangle

322. The great and small saphenous veins are the largest superficial veins of the lower limb. All of the following statements concerning the great and small saphenous veins are correct **EXCEPT**:

(A)   The great and small saphenous veins begin, respectively, as the medial and lateral extensions of the dorsal venous arch of the foot.

(B)   The small saphenous vein extends upward into the leg by passing behind the lateral malleolus.

(C)   The great saphenous vein extends upward into the leg by passing behind the medial malleolus.

(D)   The tributaries of the great saphenous vein drain all the superficial tissues of the lower limb except those of the lateral side of the foot and the posterolateral aspect of the leg.

(E)   The small saphenous vein commonly ends by uniting with the popliteal vein.

ANSWERS AND TUTORIAL ON ITEMS 319-322

The answers are: **319-B; 320-C; 321-E; 322-C**. The patient suffers from **deep venous thrombosis** (occlusion of a vein by a thrombus). In the limbs, the symptoms associated with acute venous thrombosis can vary from the absence of any symptoms to severe localized pain and evidence of systemic inflammation (such as fever, tachycardia, and anxiety). Limited collateral venous drainage may produce cyanosis of the skin. The three major predisposing factors for venous thrombosis are venous stasis, alterations in the venous wall and abnormalities in the blood coagulation system.

An **arterial embolism** the sudden obstruction of an artery by a clot or plug transported by blood flow from the heart or other blood vessel to the site of obstruction. A thrombus dislodged from a deep leg vein could be transported into the right atrium of the heart by consecutively passing through the popliteal vein, femoral vein, external iliac vein, common iliac vein, and inferior vena cava. If the embolus passed from the right atrium into the right ventricle and were ejected into the pulmonary trunk, it would finally become lodged within one of the pulmonary arteries or its branches.

There are several sites in the lower limb at which deep veins can be palpated for tenderness from venous thrombosis. The region deep to the medial aspect of the **Achilles tendon** contains the posterior tibial vein. The anterior region between the tibia and fibula in the lower leg contains the anterior tibial vein. The intramuscular veins of the soleus are a common site of deep venous thrombosis in the lower limb and these veins can be compressed by palpation of the upper part of the calf of the leg. Deep palpation of the popliteal fossa puts pressure upon the popliteal vein. In the most superior part of the femoral triangle, the femoral vein can be

161

compressed by palpation of the region immediately medial to the pulsations of the femoral artery.

The **great saphenous vein** is frequently selected for intravenous administration of fluids and medications. It ascends from the foot into the leg by passing anterior to the medial malleolus.

<u>**Items 323-325**</u>

In the following items, match each bone with its image in **Figure 3.25**.

323.   Talus

324.   Navicular

325.   Calcaneus

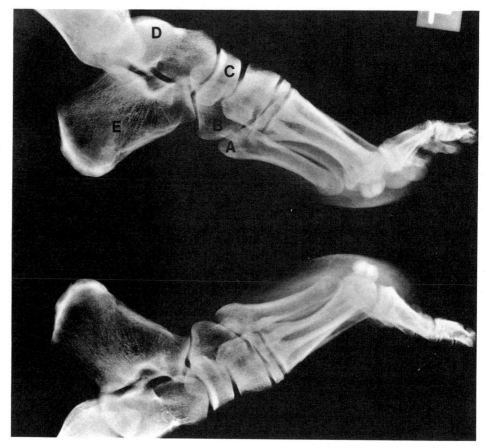

Figure 3.25

ANSWERS AND TUTORIAL ON ITEMS 323-325

The answers are: **323-D; 324-C; 325-E. Figure 3.25** is a labeled radiograph of the foot. A is the base of the **5th metatarsal.** B is the **cuboid**. The **navicular** (C) articulates with the talus posteriorly and the three cuneiform bones anteriorly. The **talus** (D) articulates with the tibia and fibula in the ankle joint. The talus forms the keystone of the medial longitudinal arch of the foot. The **calcaneus** (E) forms the heel of the foot.

Items 326-330

A 60-year-old man complaining of chest wall pain has a rash with clear vesicles with an erythematous base extending along the right 7th intercostal space. A diagnosis of herpes zoster is made based on the cutaneous distribution and appearance of the vesicular lesions.

Choose the **BEST** response.

326.   The rash is the result of reactivation of a latent viral infection of the

      (A)   intercostal arteries
      (B)   intercostal veins
      (C)   lymphatics
      (D)   intercostal muscles
      (E)   dorsal root ganglion

327.   The costal cartilage of which rib articulates with the sternum at the level of the sternal angle?

      (A)   1st
      (B)   2nd
      (C)   3rd
      (D)   4th
      (E)   5th

328. The costal cartilage of which rib is the lowest costal cartilage to contribute to the costal margin of the rib cage?

    (A)   8th
    (B)   9th
    (C)   10th
    (D)   11th
    (E)   12th

329. All of the following statements regarding the 7th intercostal nerve are correct **EXCEPT**:

    (A)   Branches innervate the skin overlying the 7th intercostal space.
    (B)   Branches innervate the parietal pleura underlying the 7th intercostal space.
    (C)   Branches innervate the skin overlying the tip of the xiphoid process.
    (D)   Branches innervate the external and internal intercostal muscles of the 7th intercostal space.
    (E)   As it extends through its intercostal space, it lies close to the upper border of the 8th rib.

330. All of the following statements regarding the intercostal arteries and veins of the 7th intercostal space are correct **EXCEPT**:

    (A)   The anterior intercostal arteries are branches of the musculophrenic artery.
    (B)   The posterior intercostal artery is a branch of the descending thoracic aorta.
    (C)   The intercostal veins drain anteriorly into the musculophrenic vein.
    (D)   The intercostal veins drain posteriorly into the azygos system of veins.
    (E)   As the intercostal arteries and veins extend through it, they lie superficial to the internal intercostal muscle.

ANSWERS AND TUTORIAL ON ITEMS 326-330

The answers are: **326-E; 327-B; 328-C; 329-E; 330-E**. The vesicular lesions of herpes zoster (shingles) are characteristically distributed throughout the dermatome of the spinal nerve with the infected dorsal root ganglion. The **sternal angle** (SA) is the posterior angle between the manubrium and the body of the sternum at the **manubriosternal joint** (MJ) (**Figure 3.26**). The manubriosternal joint can be palpated easily as a horizontal ridge in the midline of the anterior chest wall because the sternal angle is less than 180°. The costal cartilage of the 2nd rib usually articulates with the sternum at the level of the sternal angle, or manubriosternal joint (MJ) (**Figure 3.27**). Palpation of the manubriosternal joint thus permits numerical identification of the ribs. The costal cartilages of the 7th to 10th ribs form, on each side, the **costal margin** (CM) of the rib cage.

Each intercostal nerve innervates the intercostal muscles of its intercostal space and provides sensory innervation for the skin and the underlying parietal pleura. Branches of the 7th intercostal nerve also provide sensory innervation for the skin overlying the most superior part of the anterolateral abdominal wall (including the skin overlying the xiphoid process) and the underlying parietal peritoneum. Each **intercostal nerve** (N) extends through its intercostal space closely bundled with an **intercostal artery** (A) and **vein** (V) (**Figure 3.28**) and lies partially under the cover of the **costal groove** (CG) of the upper rib and directly deep to the internal intercostal muscle.

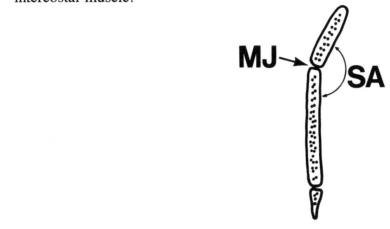

Figure 3.26

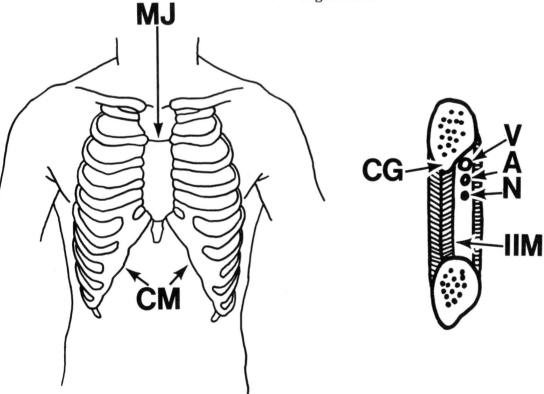

Figure 3.27

Figure 3.28

Items 331-336

The following items address information pertaining to percussing the lungs. Match the lettered area or level on each diagram with the **MOST** appropriate answer.

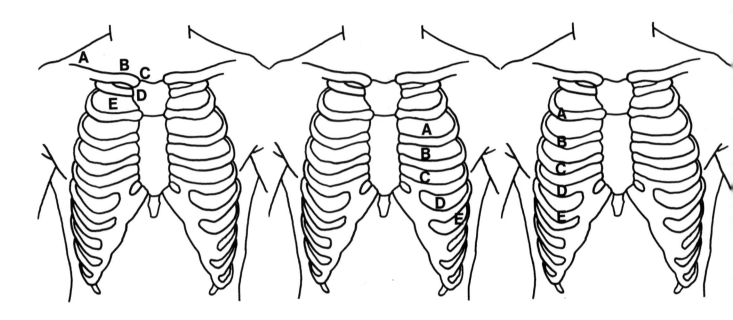

| **Figure 3.29** | **Figure 3.30** | **Figure 3.31** |

331.   Area in **Figure 3.29** where the apex of the right lung can be percussed?

332.   Area in **Figure 3.30** where the lowest part of the upper lobe of the left lung can be percussed?

333.   At midinspiration, which level in **Figure 3.31** marks the surface projection of the horizontal fissure of the right lung?

334.   Which labelled level in **Figure 3.32** of the posterior chest is the lowest area where the upper lobe of the left lung can percussed?

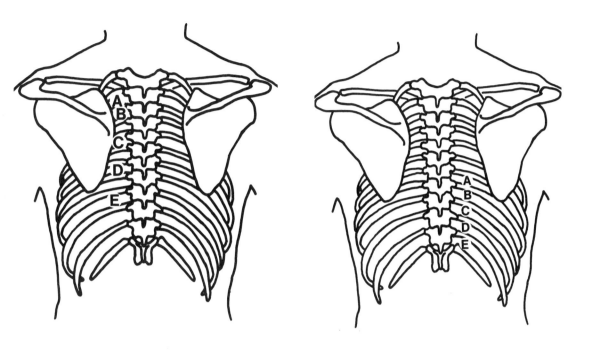

Figure 3.32   Figure 3.33

335.   At full and deep inspiration, which labelled level in **Figure 3.33** of the posterior chest wall marks the level of the costodiaphragmatic margin of the right lung?

167

336. Which labelled level in **Figure 3.34** of the lateral chest wall marks the level of the costodiaphragmatic margin of the right pleural cavity along the midaxillary line?

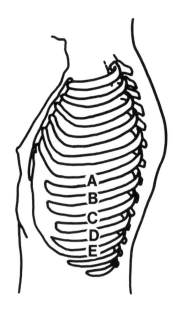

Figure 3.34

ANSWERS AND TUTORIAL ON ITEMS 331-336

The answers are: **331-B; 332-D; 333-C; 334-B; 335-E; 336-E**. The bony and cartilaginous parts of the rib cage can serve to mark the surface projections of the pleural cavities and the lobes of the lungs. The most important surface relationships are as follows:

(1) The apex (A) of each lung projects above the medial third of the clavicle (**Figure 3.35**).

(2) For both lungs, the surface projection of the oblique fissure (OF) is an arc which begins posteriorly between the tips of the spinous processes of the 4th and 5th thoracic vertebrae, crosses the 5th and 6th ribs as it extends laterally to the midaxillary line, and then overlaps the lower border of the 6th rib to the lateral border of the sternum (**Figure 3.35** and **Figure 3.36**).

(3) For the right lung, the surface projection of the horizontal fissure (HF) is an arc which overlaps the lower border of the 4th rib from the midaxillary line to the lateral border of the sternum (**Figures 3.35**).

The **costodiaphragmatic margin** (CMP) of each pleural cavity lies at the level of the 8th rib at the midclavicular line, the 10th rib at the midaxillary line, and the 11th or 12th rib at the lateral border of the vertebral column. At midinspiration, the costodiaphragmatic margin of each lung (CML) lies 2 rib spaces above the costodiaphragmatic margin of its pleural cavity (**Figures 3.35** and **3.36**). The costodiaphragmatic margin of each lung descends inferiorly to the costodiaphragmatic margin of its pleural cavity at full and deep inspiration.

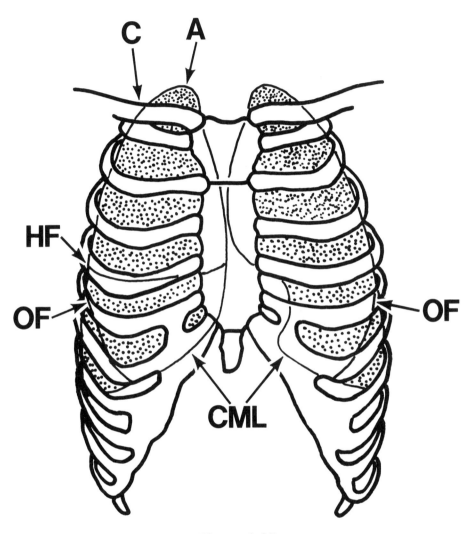

Figure 3.35

169

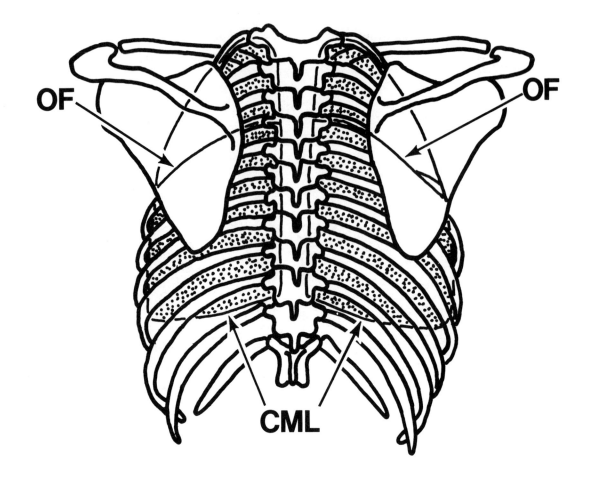

Figure 3.36

170

During a routine physical examination, an asymptomatic, 22-year-old woman presents with a midsystolic click followed by a late systolic crescendo-type murmur. Echocardiography shows a prolapsing posterior leaflet of the mitral valve.

Choose the **BEST** response.

337. Which of the labeled positions in **Figure 3.37** is the **BEST** site for hearing the heart murmur?

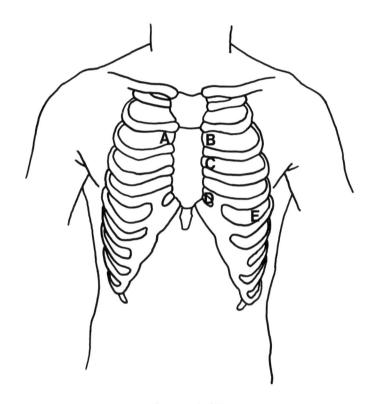

Figure 3.37

338. Certain procedures commonly move the late systolic murmur of a prolapsing mitral valve either toward or away from S1 (the first heart sound). All of the following statements concerning these procedures are correct **EXCEPT**:

(A) Administration of a vasodilator should move the murmur away from S1.
(B) Moving from a supine to a standing position should move the murmur toward S1.
(C) Squatting should move the murmur away from S1.
(D) Exertion of the Valsalva maneuver should move the murmur toward S1.
(E) Making tight fists with the hands should move the murmur away from S1.

339. The first heart sound has two components because it is produced by the near-simultaneous closure of two valves. These two valves are the

   (A)   tricuspid and pulmonary valves
   (B)   mitral and aortic valves
   (C)   aortic and pulmonary valves
   (D)   tricuspid and mitral valves
   (E)   pulmonary and mitral valves

ANSWERS AND TUTORIAL ON ITEMS 337-339

The answers are: **337-E; 338-A; 339-D**. The best site for hearing the closure of the **mitral valve** is the site in the **left 5th intercostal space** where the apex of the heart beats against the anterior chest wall during systole. This site is generally also the best site for hearing the murmur produced by a prolapsing mitral valve.

In persons with a prolapsing mitral valve, prolapse does not generally occur until midsystole. It is believed that the **midsystolic click** emanates from the prolapsed mitral valve leaflet or its chordae tendinea when they are acutely tensed at the moment of maximum prolapse. Regurgitation of blood from the left ventricle into the left atrium through the prolapsed mitral valve generates the late systolic murmur. Procedures which decrease systemic venous return to the heart (administration of a vasodilator, moving from a supine to a standing position, or exertion of the **Valsalva maneuver**) decrease left ventricular end-diastolic volume and thus move the click and murmur toward S1. By contrast, procedures which increase systemic venous return to the heart (squatting or isometric exercises) increase left ventricular end-diastolic volume and thus delay the onset of the click and murmur.

The beginning of **systole** during the cardiac cycle is marked by ventricular contraction concurring with atrial relaxation. These concurrent events on both sides of the heart promptly generate a blood pressure in each contracting ventricle which exceeds that in the adjoining, relaxing atrium. This pressure difference across each atrioventricular valve closes the valve. The mitral and tricuspid valves close almost simultaneously, producing audible vibrations in the blood confined to the ventricular chambers. Collectively, the vibrations form S1, the first heart sound (the 'lub') of each heartbeat. The closure of the mitral valve slightly precedes the closure of the tricuspid valve.

Items 340-344

A 42-year-old man enters the emergency department complaining of shortness of breath and severe chest pain. The physical findings suggest pericardial tamponade. An ECG showing total electrical alternans and an echocardiogram showing pericardial effusion confirm the diagnosis.

Choose the **BEST** response.

340. All of the following physical findings are commonly encountered in cases of pericardial tamponade **EXCEPT**:

   (A) shift of the right border of cardiac dullness to the right
   (B) sinus tachycardia
   (C) bilateral distension of the jugular veins
   (D) increased intensity of S1 and S2
   (E) decrease of the systolic blood pressure

341. Which jugular vein is commonly the **BEST** barometer of central venous pressure?

   (A) right anterior
   (B) right external
   (C) right internal
   (D) left external
   (E) left internal

342. All of the following statements concerning the jugular, subclavian and brachiocephalic veins are correct **EXCEPT**:

   (A) The anterior jugular ends via union with either the external jugular or subclavian.
   (B) The internal jugular ends at its union with the subclavian.
   (C) The union of the external jugular with the subclavian forms the brachiocephalic.
   (D) The union of the left and right brachiocephalic forms the superior vena cava.
   (E) In the mediastinum, the right brachiocephalic is more vertical than the left brachiocephalic.

343. If the head, neck, and trunk of a supine adult are elevated 30-45°, what is the normal vertical distance above the level of the sternal angle that pulsatile activity will be observed in the jugular veins?

   (A) 0-1 cm
   (B) 2-3 cm
   (C) 4-5 cm
   (D) 6-7 cm
   (E) 8-9 cm

344. In a normal, healthy adult, the right border of the heart lies to the right of the right border of the sternum by

    (A)   0-2 cm
    (B)   2-4 cm
    (C)   4-6 cm
    (D)   6-8 cm
    (E)   8-10 cm

ANSWERS AND TUTORIAL ON ITEMS 340-344

The answers are: **340-D; 341-C; 342-C; 343-B; 344-A**. **Pericardial tamponade** (excess fluid in the pericardial cavity) broadens the region of cardiac dullness in the anterior chest wall, shifting it to the right from its normal location about 1 cm to the right of the right sternal border. The pressure exerted by the pericardial fluid decreases intracardiac diastolic pressures, and thereby reduces venous return to the right atrium (as evidenced by bilateral distension of jugular veins) and systolic blood pressure. Sinus tachycardia occurs as a compensatory mechanism to maintain cardiac output. Pericardial tamponade also diminishes the intensity of S1 and S2.

The **internal** and **external jugular** (IJ and EJ), **subclavian** (S), and **brachiocephalic** (B) **veins** and **superior vena cava** (SVC) are the major venous trunks which extend through the neck and superior mediastinum to conduct blood into the right atrium (**Figure 3.38**). When a normal adult is standing or seated upright, blood fills these venous trunks to a level about 2-3 cm above the sternal angle, i.e., blood fills the superior vena cava, brachiocephalic veins, and subclavian veins completely but only the lower parts of the jugular veins. The height to which the jugular veins are filled is proportional to right atrial pressure. Accordingly, the jugular veins can serve as manometers of right atrial pressure. Right atrial pressure is frequently called **central venous pressure** (CVP), since the blood pressure of the right atrium approximates that of the large systemic veins converging upon the right atrium.

The **right internal jugular vein** is the most appropriate jugular vein to select for the measurement of CVP because it is the only jugular vein which forms a straight continuation with the right brachiocephalic vein and superior vena cava (**Figure 3.38**). The angular unions of the left internal jugular vein with the left brachiocephalic vein and of the external jugular veins with the subclavian veins makes their blood heights less reliable monitors of CVP.

174

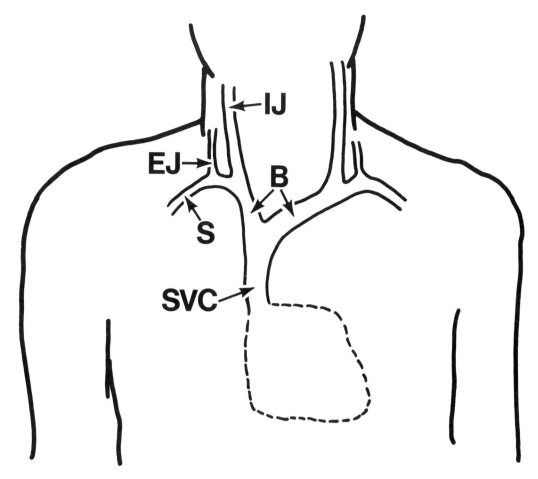

Figure 3.38

During each heartbeat, there are three pulsatile increases in right atrial pressure. The first increase (the **a wave**) coincides with atrial contraction. The second increase (the **c wave**) occurs during early systole, when increasing pressure in the right ventricle bulges the tricuspid valve into the right atrium. The third increase (the **v wave**) occurs as blood flows into the right atrium during late systole. These increases are transmitted in a retrograde fashion through the blood in the internal and external jugular veins. When these jugular venous pulses reach the meniscus (curved, upper surface) of the blood in each jugular vein, they produce fluctuations in the level of the meniscus, and thus pulsations of the overlying skin. These cutaneous jugular pulses are the best indicator of the height to which blood fills the veins.

Inspection of **jugular pulses** should begin with the patient in the supine position. In a normal individual, the jugular veins will be distended because the jugular veins and the right atrium now are all at about the same level. The patient's head, neck, and trunk are next elevated sufficiently to lower the height of the jugular pulses to a level which is below the angle of the mandible but above the clavicle (a 30-45° elevation is generally sufficient). In a normal adult, pulsatile activity will be visible near the lower ends of the jugular veins, commonly up to a vertical distance of 2-3 cm above the level of the sternal angle. This is because the average CVP in a normal individual is about 7-8 cm water, and the center of the right atrium is about 5 cm below the level of the sternal angle.

A 63-year-old woman enters the emergency department complaining of chest pain and fainting after exertion. The physical findings (one of which is an ejection murmur) suggest severe aortic stenosis. An ECG showing left ventricular hypertrophy and an echocardiogram showing a thickened, calcified aortic valve confirm the diagnosis.

Choose the **BEST** response.

345.   All of the following physical findings are commonly encountered in cases of severe aortic stenosis **EXCEPT**:

    (A)   diminished intensity of S2
    (B)   slow-rising carotid arterial upstrokes
    (C)   radiation of the ejection murmur to the carotid arteries
    (D)   shift of the apical thrust upward and laterally
    (E)   marked precordial apical thrust

346.   The second heart sound has two components because it is produced by the nearly simultaneous closure of two valves. These two valves are the

    (A)   aortic and pulmonary
    (B)   tricuspid and mitral
    (C)   aortic and mitral
    (D)   pulmonary and mitral
    (E)   aortic and tricuspid

347.   The apex beat (point of maximum impulse, PMI) is normally found

    (A)   7-9 cm to the left of the midsternal line in the 3rd intercostal space
    (B)   7-9 cm to the left of the midsternal line in the 5th intercostal space
    (C)   7-9 cm to the left of the midsternal line in the 7th intercostal space
    (D)   7-9 cm to the left of the midsternal line in the 9th intercostal space
    (E)   7-9 cm to the left of the midsternal line in the 11th intercostal space

348. Which of the labelled positions in **Figure 3.39** is the **BEST** site for hearing the closure of the aortic valve?

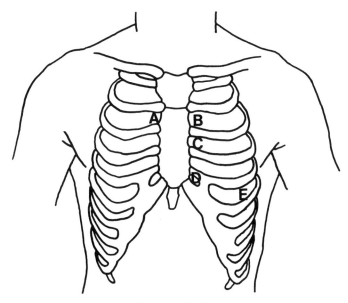

Figure 3.39

ANSWERS AND TUTORIAL ON ITEMS 345-348

The answers are: **345-D; 346-A; 347-C; 348-A**. In this case, **aortic stenosis** is the result of progressive calcification of the aortic valve leaflets. Left ventricular hypertrophy has served to maintain left ventricular output. A stenosed aortic valve restricts and disturbs left ventricular outflow during **systole**. The restriction prolongs ejection and thus delays the attainment of peak carotid pressure. The disturbance of left ventricular outflow produces an **ejection murmur** that is transmitted in an antegrade fashion to the carotid arteries. The intensity of the sound produced by the closure of the aortic valve at the end of systole is diminished because the valve leaflets are thick and stiff. The contraction of the hypertrophic left ventricle produces the marked **precordial apical thrust**. Left ventricular hypertrophy shifts the apex of the heart, and thus the PMI, downward and laterally. The **exertional angina** is due to insufficient blood supply to the hypertrophic left ventricle. Such insufficiency can occur with even unobstructed coronary arteries. The **exertional syncope** (fainting) is due to inadequate cerebral perfusion.

Toward the end of systole, after the ventricles have ejected most of their blood, retrograde flow of blood from the pulmonary trunk and aorta into the ventricles begins as a consequence of the blood pressure in each arterial trunk being greater than that in the ventricle. This retrograde blood flow snaps the pulmonary and aortic valves shut. Their nearly simultaneous closure generates audible vibrations in the blood borne by both arterial trunks. Collectively, these vibrations produce the second heart sound (the 'dup') of the heartbeat. The closure of the aortic valve precedes the closure of the pulmonary valve during inspiration.

A 34-year-old woman makes an appointment with a primary care physician because of recent exertional chest pain. The physical and radiographic findings suggest advanced primary pulmonary hypertension.

Choose the **BEST** response.

349.   All of the following findings are consistent with this diagnosis **EXCEPT**:

      (A)   a palpable parasternal heave
      (B)   diminished intensity of the pulmonic component of S2
      (C)   a PA chest film showing enlarged pulmonary arteries
      (D)   shift of the apical thrust upward and laterally
      (E)   increased jugular venous pressure

350.   Which of the positions in **Figure 3.40** is the **BEST** site for hearing the closure of the pulmonary valve?

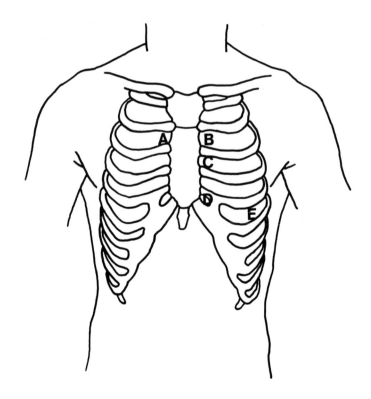

Figure 3.40

351. All of the following statements concerning the bronchial arteries and veins of the lungs are correct **EXCEPT**:

    (A)   The root of the lung transmits the bronchial arteries into the lung and the bronchial vein out of the lung.

    (B)   The bronchial vein drains the capillary beds of the conducting airways of the lung.

    (C)   The azygos system of veins commonly drains the bronchial veins.

    (D)   The bronchial arteries supply the conducting airways.

    (E)   The bronchial arteries are branches of the aortic arch.

ANSWERS AND TUTORIAL ON ITEMS 349-351

The answers are: **349-B; 350-B; 351-E**. **Primary pulmonary hypertension** is a disease in which the resistance to pulmonary blood flow markedly increases as a result of smooth muscle hypertrophy and intimal proliferation of the pulmonary arteries and arterioles. Right ventricular output in initially maintained by **right ventricular hypertrophy**. Contraction of the hypertrophic right ventricle produces a palpable, **parasternal heave**. Right ventricular hypertrophy also shifts the apex of the heart, and thus the PMI, upward and laterally. The significant elevation of pulmonary arterial pressure enlarges the pulmonary arteries and results in a more forceful closure of the pulmonic valve leaflets at the end of systole (thus producing a louder pulmonic component in S2). The inadequacy of right ventricular function in advanced cases leads to venous congestion and a rise in CVP and thus elevated jugular venous pressure. Distension of the pulmonary arteries or their major branches is the basis of the patient's **exertional chest pain**. Each lung is supplied by one or two **bronchial arteries**. These arteries arise from either the descending thoracic aorta or the upper posterior intercostal arteries.

A 37-year-old woman makes an appointment with a cardiologist because of the inefficacy of her medication in managing unstable angina. The cardiologist recommends coronary arteriography to see if she would benefit from revascularization. In the following items, match each coronary artery or arterial branch with its image in **Figure 3.41**.

352. Left anterior descending artery (anterior interventricular branch of the left coronary artery)

353. Right coronary artery

354. Posterior descending artery (posterior interventricular branch of the right coronary artery)

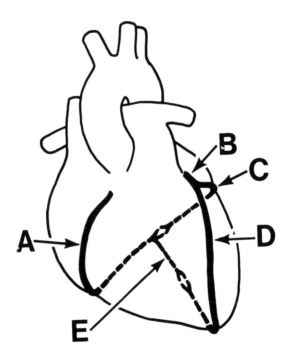

Figure 3.41

In the following items, match each cardiac vein with its image in **Figure 3.42** below, a view of the sternocostal surface of the heart.

355.   Middle cardiac vein

356.   Coronary sinus

357.   Great cardiac vein

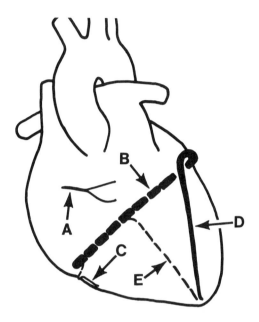

Figure 3.42

ANSWERS AND TUTORIAL ON ITEMS 352-357

The answers are: **352-D; 353-A; 354-E; 355-E; 356-B; 357-D. Figures 3.41** (arteries) and **3.42** (veins) are sternocostal views of the heart. In **Figure 3.41**, B is the **left coronary artery** and C is the **circumflex artery**. In **Figure 3.42**, A is an **anterior cardiac vein** and C is the **small cardiac vein**.

In the following items, match each structure with an image of one of its borders in the labelled PA radiograph of the chest in **Figure 3.43**.

358.   Aortic arch (aortic knob)

359.   Pulmonary trunk

360.   Left ventricle

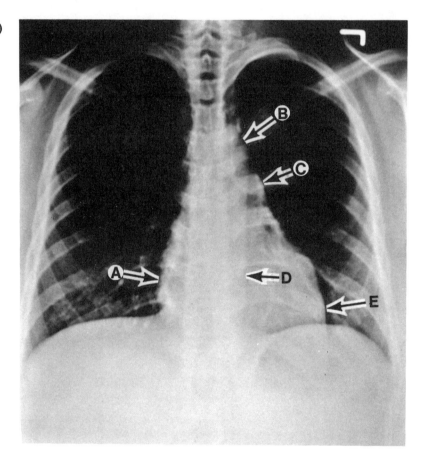

Figure 3.43

ANSWERS AND TUTORIAL ON ITEMS 358-360

The answers are: **358-B; 359-C; 360-E**. A is the right border of the **right atrium**, B is the aortic arch (aortic knuckle or knob), C is the pulmonary trunk, D is the left border of the **descending thoracic aorta** and E is the left ventricle.

The three CT scans in **Figure 3.44** are adjacent 10 mm-thick scans of the thorax. In the following items, match each structure with its image in the labeled CT scan.

361.   Right brachiocephalic vein

362.   Brachiocephalic trunk

363.   Left common carotid artery

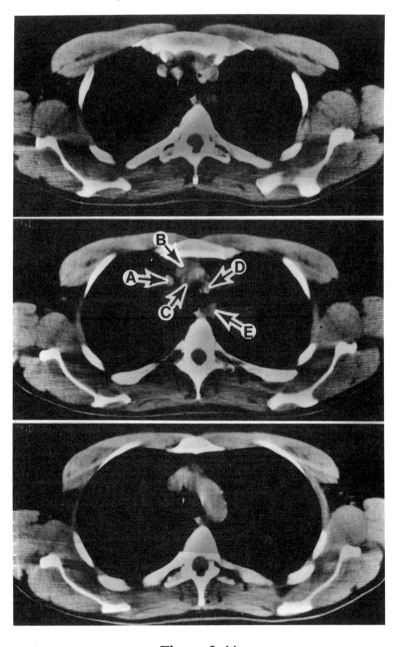

Figure 3.44

The answers are: **361-A; 362-C; 363-D**. B is the **left brachiocephalic vein**, and E is the **left subclavian artery**.

The middle CT scan displays the blood vessels in the **mediastinum** above the level of the aortic arch. The vessels include the three branches of the aortic arch (which, in the order of their origin, are the brachiocephalic trunk, left common carotid artery, and left subclavian artery) and the two veins (the left and right brachiocephalic veins) that join to form the superior vena cava. The brachiocephalic trunk divides to form the right common carotid and right subclavian arteries.

Items 364-370

The eight CT scans in **Figure 3.45** are adjacent 10 mm-thick scans of the thorax. In the following items, match each structure with its image in the labelled CT scans.

364. Right atrium

365. Left atrium

366. Left brachiocephalic vein

367. Right pulmonary artery

368. Ascending aorta

369. Esophagus

370. Left main stem (primary) bronchus

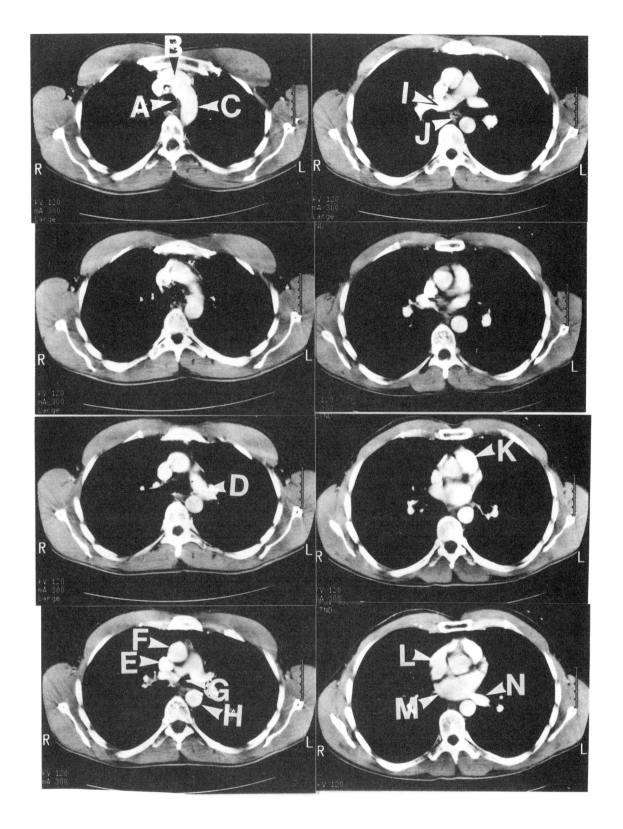

Figure 3.45

ANSWERS AND TUTORIAL ON ITEMS 364-370

The answers are: **364-L; 365-M; 366-B; 367-I; 368-F; 369-J; 370-G**. A is the **trachea**, C is the **aortic arch**, D is the **left pulmonary artery**, E is the **superior vena cava**, H is the **descending thoracic aorta**, K is the **pulmonary trunk**, and N is a **left pulmonary vein**. The eight CT scans display the thorax from the level of the aortic arch (the first scan) down to the level of the left atrium (the last scan). The first scan shows the **aortic arch** extending posteriorly as it passes to the left of the trachea. The left brachiocephalic vein extends rightward to join the right brachiocephalic vein. The second scan skirts the undersurface of the aortic arch. At this level, the trachea widens to divide into the left and right main stem bronchi.

The third scan shows the **carina** (the keel-like ridge between the main stem bronchi) and the left pulmonary artery. Observe that as the left pulmonary artery extends leftward between the ascending aorta and descending thoracic aorta, it passes directly inferior to the aortic arch.

The fourth scans lies at the level at which the left and right pulmonary arteries arise from the pulmonary trunk. The superior vena cava lies to the right and posterior to the ascending aorta. The descending thoracic aorta lies to the left of a thoracic vertebral body.

The fifth scan shows the right pulmonary artery extending toward the right lung. The scans in this series are typical in that the level at which the left pulmonary artery is best visualized (the level of the third scan) is superior to that at which the right pulmonary artery is best visualized (the level of the fifth scan). The fifth scan also features the esophagus lying directly anterior to and just slightly to the left of the vertebral column.

The seventh scan extends through the upper part of the left atrium. The pulmonary trunk ascends to the left of the ascending aorta.

The eighth scan extends through both the left and right atria and shows a left pulmonary vein joining the left atrium.

Items 371-377

A helpful way to understand the organization of the abdomen and pelvis is to visualize, in the order shown, the placement of the following five groups of organs:

[1]   The retroperitoneal viscera of the abdomen
[2]   The secondarily retroperitoneal viscera of the abdomen
[3]   The intraperitoneal segments of the small and large intestines in the mid and lower abdomen
[4]   The liver and gallbladder and the intraperitoneal viscera in the upper abdomen, and
[5]   The pelvic viscera

The following items review the peritoneal relationships among abdominal and pelvic viscera.

Choose the **BEST** response.

371.   All of the following viscera are retroperitoneal **EXCEPT**:

(A)   abdominal aorta
(B)   spleen
(C)   right kidney
(D)   left adrenal gland
(E)   inferior vena cava

372.   All of the following viscera are secondarily retroperitoneal **EXCEPT**:

(A)   ascending colon
(B)   head of the pancreas
(C)   body of the pancreas
(D)   tail of the pancreas
(E)   descending colon

373.   All of the following viscera are intraperitoneal **EXCEPT**:

(A)   2nd, 3rd, and 4th parts of the duodenum
(B)   jejunum
(C)   ileum
(D)   transverse colon
(E)   sigmoid colon

374. All of the following regions are located in the greater sac **EXCEPT**:

   (A)   region anterior to the mesentery of the small intestine
   (B)   left lateral paracolic gutter
   (C)   hepatorenal recess (Morrison's pouch)
   (D)   region posterior to the stomach
   (E)   rectouterine pouch (pouch of Douglas)

375. All of the following statements regarding the epiploic foramen are correct **EXCEPT**:

   (A)   It is a passageway between the greater and lesser sacs of the peritoneal cavity.
   (B)   A part of the caudate lobe of the liver borders it superiorly.
   (C)   The proximal half of the 1st part of the duodenum borders it inferiorly.
   (D)   The portal vein borders it posteriorly.
   (E)   The free right margin of the lesser omentum borders it anteriorly.

376. All of the following peritoneal ligaments border (line) a part of the lesser sac **EXCEPT**:

   (A)   lesser omentum
   (B)   splenorenal ligament
   (C)   gastrophrenic ligament
   (D)   gastrocolic ligament
   (E)   falciform ligament

377. All of the following statements are correct **EXCEPT**:

   (A)   The fundus of the uterus is covered with peritoneum.
   (B)   In the midline, the peritoneum which covers the anterior surface of the middle third of the rectum is continuous anteriorly with the peritoneum that covers the uppermost posterior surface of the vagina.
   (C)   In the midline, the peritoneum which covers the anterior surface of the uterus is continuous anteriorly with the peritoneum that covers the uppermost anterior surface of the vagina.
   (D)   The superior surface of the urinary bladder is covered with peritoneum.
   (E)   The ovary is attached by the mesovarium to the posterior peritoneum layer of the broad ligament of the uterus.

The answers are: **371-B; 372-D; 373-A; 374-D; 375-D; 376-E; 377-C**. The **retroperitoneal viscera** of the abdomen include the abdominal aorta, inferior vena cava, kidneys, adrenal glands, and ureters. The spleen is intraperitoneal. The **secondarily retroperitoneal viscera** of the abdomen include the head, neck, and body of the pancreas; the distal half of the 1st part of the duodenum and the 2nd, 3rd, and 4th parts of the duodenum; the ascending colon with the hepatic flexure at the upper end; and the descending colon with the splenic flexure at the upper end. The tail of the pancreas is intraperitoneal, lying sandwiched between the two peritoneum layers of the splenorenal ligament.

The **lesser sac** of the peritoneal cavity is sealed off superiorly by the diaphragm, anteriorly by the lesser omentum, stomach and gastrocolic ligament, inferiorly by the transverse colon and transverse mesocolon, posteriorly by the upper posterior abdominal wall, and on the left by the gastrophrenic, gastrosplenic, and splenorenal ligaments.

On the right, the lesser sac communicates with the greater sac via a passageway called the **epiploic foramen.** The epiploic foramen is the only passageway between the greater and lesser sacs and has four borders:

- The caudate process of the caudate lobe of the liver borders the foramen superiorly.
- The free right margin of the lesser omentum borders the foramen anteriorly and transmits the portal vein, hepatic artery proper, and bile duct.
- The proximal half of the 1st part of the duodenum borders the foramen inferiorly.
- The inferior vena cava borders the foramen posteriorly.

In the midline region, the **peritoneum** which covers the anterior surface of the uterus (U) is continuous anteriorly with the peritoneum that covers the superior surface of the urinary bladder (UB) (**Figure 3.46**).

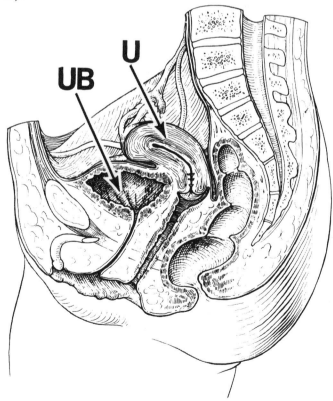

Figure 3.46

189

A loop of ileum becomes entrapped in the right inguinal canal of a 10-year-old boy who has had a patent processes vaginalis in the right inguinal canal since birth.

Choose the **BEST** response.

378. Visceral pain from the entrapped ileal loop will **MOST** likely be felt in the

    (A)   epigastric region
    (B)   umbilical region
    (C)   hypogastric region
    (D)   right inguinal region
    (E)   right lumbar region

379. Sensory fibers from the jejunum, ileum, and cecum enter the spinal cord at spinal cord segment levels

    (A)   C3, C4, and C5
    (B)   T5, T6, T7, T8, and T9
    (C)   T8, T9, T10, T11, and T12
    (D)   T10, T11, T12, L1, and L2
    (E)   L1, L2, S2, S3, and S4

380. All of the following statements concerning abdominal hernias are correct **EXCEPT**:

    (A)   The neck of the sac of a femoral hernia always lies immediately medial and superior to the pubic tubercle.
    (B)   The neck of the sac of an indirect inguinal hernia always lies lateral to the inferior epigastric artery.
    (C)   The neck of the sac of a direct inguinal hernia always lies medial to the origin of the inferior epigastric artery.
    (D)   The sac of a hernia consists of an outpouching of parietal peritoneum.
    (E)   The neck of the sac of a hernia is the proximal end of the sac.

381. All of the following statements concerning the inguinal canal are correct **EXCEPT**:

(A) The external spermatic fascia is continuous with the aponeurotic tendon of external oblique at the superficial inguinal ring.

(B) The internal spermatic fascia is continuous with the transversalis fascia at the deep inguinal ring.

(C) The aponeurotic tendon of external oblique forms most of the anterior wall of the inguinal canal.

(D) The inguinal ligament forms the floor of the inguinal canal.

(E) Transversalis fascia forms most of the roof of the inguinal canal.

ANSWERS AND TUTORIAL ON ITEMS 378-381

The answers are: **378-B; 379-C; 380-A; 381-E. Visceral pain** is a dull, sickening pain that is poorly localized to one of the midline regions (epigastric, umbilical, or hypogastric) of the abdomen. Visceral pain is produced by the stimulation of visceral pain fibers which are sensitive to acute stretching and anoxia. Disease or injury of the abdominal viscera supplied by the superior mesenteric artery (which include the ileum) produces visceral pain that is most commonly localized to the **umbilical region**.

The greater, lesser, and least splanchnic nerves provide almost all the preganglionic sympathetic innervation for the viscera supplied by the superior mesenteric artery. The sensory fibers that innervate the viscera supplied by the superior mesenteric artery enter the spinal cord at those spinal cord segments that provide preganglionic sympathetic innervation for the viscera (specifically, the sensory fibers enter at the T8-T12 levels).

Indirect inguinal hernia occurs when viscera protrude into the inguinal canal through the deep inguinal ring (DIR) (**Figure 3.47**). The neck of the sac of an indirect inguinal hernia thus always lies lateral to the inferior epigastric artery (IEA). An indirect inguinal hernia usually results because of a patent processus vaginalis, a derivative of the parietal peritoneum.

Direct inguinal hernia occurs when the peritoneum or viscera protrude into the inguinal canal through a distention of its posterior wall. The neck of the sac of a direct inguinal hernia lies medial to the origin of the inferior epigastric artery and within the inguinal (Hesselbach's) triangle. The inguinal triangle is the area within the inguinal region bounded by the inferior epigastric artery (IEA) laterally, the lateral edge of rectus abdominis (RA) medially, and the inguinal ligament (IG) inferiorly (**Figure 3.47**).

Femoral hernia occurs when the peritoneum or viscera protrude through the femoral ring (FR) into the femoral canal (**Figure 3.47**). The neck of the sac of a femoral hernia always lies immediately lateral and inferior to the pubic tubercle (PT). The lower free borders of internal oblique and transversus abdominis form the roof of the inguinal canal.

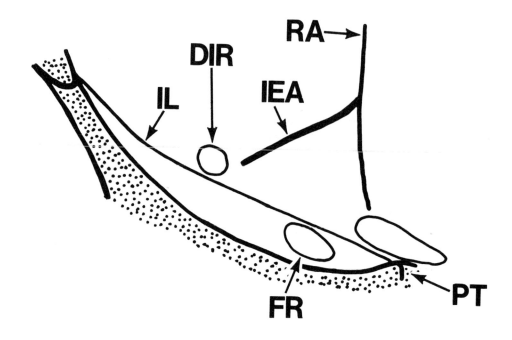

Figure 3.47

A 49-year-old woman has had upper abdominal pain for the last 5 days. Her symptoms include pain typical of biliary colic, intermittent fevers with chills, yellowish sclera and oral mucosa, a tender gallbladder, and an enlarged and tender liver. A diagnosis of ascending cholangitis (ascending sepsis of the extrahepatic and intrahepatic biliary ducts and the gallbladder) is made on the basis of the history and physical exam. Upon admission to a hospital, ultrasound examination of the patient's biliary tract shows gallstones in the lumen of the gallbladder, dilated intrahepatic biliary ducts, and a gallstone lodged in the lower part of the common bile duct.

Choose the **BEST** response.

382. Visceral pain from the biliary ducts is **MOST** likely referred to which abdominal region?

    (A)   epigastric
    (B)   umbilical
    (C)   hypogastric
    (D)   right lumbar
    (E)   right inguinal

383. Disease of the biliary ducts may produce referred pain in all of the following cutaneous regions **EXCEPT**:

   (A)   point of the shoulder
   (B)   right upper quadrant of the anterolateral abdominal wall
   (C)   anterior chest wall overlying the 6th, 7th, and 8th intercostal spaces
   (D)   posterior chest wall overlying the inferior angle of the scapula
   (E)   posterior chest wall overlying the medial end of the spine of the scapula

384. Which set of spinal nerves innervates the skin in the center of the right upper quadrant of the anterolateral abdominal wall?

   (A)   T4, T5, and T6
   (B)   T7, T8, and T9
   (C)   T10, T11, and T12
   (D)   L1 and L2
   (E)   L3 and L4

385. Percussion of the anterior chest and abdominal walls can be used to assess the height of the liver along the right midclavicular line. The normal range for the height of the liver in an adult is

   (A)   3-6 cm
   (B)   6-9 cm
   (C)   9-12 cm
   (D)   3-9 cm
   (E)   6-12 cm

386. All of the following statements concerning the blood supply and venous drainage of the liver are correct **EXCEPT**:

   (A)   The right hepatic artery supplies all of the caudate lobe of the liver.
   (B)   The left hepatic artery supplies all of the quadrate lobe of the liver.
   (C)   The hepatic veins drain the blood conducted to the liver by the portal vein.
   (D)   The hepatic veins drain the blood conducted to the liver by the left and right hepatic arteries.
   (E)   The hepatic veins are tributaries of the inferior vena cava.

387. All of the following statements concerning arteries that arise directly or indirectly from the celiac artery are correct **EXCEPT**:

(A)   Branches of the left gastric artery supply the stomach along the upper part of its lesser curvature.

(B)   Branches of the splenic artery supply the body and tail of the pancreas.

(C)   The left gastroepiploic artery arises from the splenic artery.

(D)   The gastroduodenal artery lies directly anterior to the first part of the duodenum.

(E)   Branches of the right gastroepiploic artery supply the stomach along the lower part of its greater curvature.

388. Portal-systemic anastomoses occur in all of the following regions **EXCEPT**:

(A)   between the middle and lower thirds of the esophagus

(B)   between the upper and lower halves of the anal canal

(C)   between the upper and lower halves of the ureter

(D)   paraumbilical region of the anterolateral abdominal wall

(E)   retroperitoneal region deep to the posterior abdominal wall

ANSWERS AND TUTORIAL ON ITEMS 382-388

The answers are: **382-A; 383-E; 384-B; 385-E; 386-A; 387-D; 388-C**. Disease or injury of the abdominal viscera supplied by the **celiac artery** (which include the liver and gallbladder) produces **visceral pain** that is most commonly localized to the **epigastric region**. The left and right **greater splanchnic nerves** provide almost all the preganglionic sympathetic innervation for the viscera supplied by the celiac artery. Almost all the sensory fibers that innervate the viscera supplied by the celiac artery enter the spinal cord at those spinal cord segments that give rise to the preganglionic sympathetic fibers for the greater splanchnic nerves (specifically, the sensory fibers enter at the T5-T9 levels). The only exceptions are some sensory fibers from the liver, gallbladder, and the extrahepatic biliary ducts that enter the spinal cord at the C3-C5 segments; the right phrenic nerve transmits these fibers to their cell bodies in the dorsal root ganglia of spinal nerves C3, C4, and C5.

Disease or injury of any of the viscera supplied by the **celiac artery** may refer pain to parts of the T5-T9 dermatomes. Of the last four cutaneous regions listed in Item 384, the right upper quadrant of the anterolateral abdominal wall represents part of the T7-T10 dermatomes, the anterior chest wall overlying the 6th, 7th, and 8th intercostal spaces represents part of the T6-T8 dermatomes, the posterior chest wall overlying the inferior angle of the scapula represents part of the T7 dermatome, and the posterior chest wall overlying the medial end of the spine of the scapula represents part of the T3 dermatome. Disease or injury of the liver, gallbladder, and extrahepatic ducts may also refer pain to the shoulder (as it represents parts of the C3-C5 dermatomes).

Percussion can be used during a physical exam to assess the size of the **liver**. As the patient lies supine and holds the breath at full expiration, the examiner percusses the anterior chest wall and anterolateral abdominal wall from the right 2nd intercostal space downward along the right midclavicular line. In a normal adult, percussion resonance (due to percussion of the right lung) is encountered down to the highest level (which is typically that of the 4th intercostal space) at which the liver crosses the right midclavicular line. A thin wedge of the right lung's lower lobe anteriorly covers the diaphragm and the underlying liver down to the level of the 6th rib; percussion of both the right lung and the liver between the levels of the 4th intercostal space and the 6th rib produces a zone of percussion dullness called hepatic dullness. A zone of percussion flatness called **hepatic flatness** is generally encountered from the level of the 6th rib down to that of the liver's anteroinferior margin. Percussion of bowel segments inferior to the liver produce **percussion dullness, resonance,** or **tympany** below the zone of hepatic flatness. The combined heights of the zones of hepatic dullness and hepatic flatness are a measure of the size of the liver; the normal range for the combined heights in an adult is 6-12 cm. It should be noted, however, that the presence of gas-filled bowel segments immediately posterior to the lower part of the liver's visceral surface can obscure determination of the lower limit of the zone of hepatic flatness, and thus lead to a faulty underestimate of liver size.

The left **hepatic artery** supplies the liver's left lobe, quadrate lobe, and caudate lobe (except for the latter's caudate process). The right hepatic artery supplies all the liver's parenchyma not supplied by the left hepatic artery. **Figure 3.48** shows the relationships of the left gastric artery (LGA), splenic artery (SA), left gastroepiploic artery (LGEA), gastroduodenal artery (GA), and right gastroepiploic artery (RGEA) to the stomach (S), pancreas (P), and 1st part of the duodenum (D). The gastroduodenal artery passes behind the first part of the duodenum before giving rise to the right gastroepiploic and superior pancreaticoduodenal arteries.

Portal-systemic anastomoses are anastomoses between veins that are tributaries of the **portal vein** and tributaries of the superior vena cava or inferior vena cava. At the junction between the middle and lower thirds of the esophagus, tributaries of the left gastric vein (which drains toward the portal vein) anastomose with tributaries of the azygos system of veins (which drains toward the superior vena cava). At the junction between the upper and lower halves of the anal canal, tributaries of the superior rectal vein (which drains toward the portal vein) anastomose with tributaries of the inferior rectal vein (which drains toward the inferior vena cava). In the paraumbilical region, tributaries of the paraumbilical veins (which drain toward the portal vein) anastomose with tributaries of the lumbar veins (which drain toward the inferior vena cava). In the retroperitoneal region deep to the posterior abdominal wall, tributaries of the splenic vein (which drains toward the portal vein) anastomoses with tributaries of the left renal vein (which drains toward the inferior vena cava).

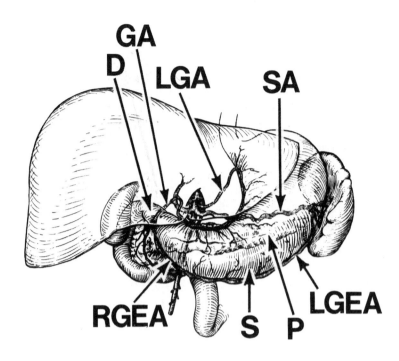

Figure 3.48

<u>Items 389-391</u>

A 16-year old girl complains of abdominal pain, nausea, and lack of appetite during the last 12 hours. She has a low grade fever (101.0° F). A tentative diagnosis of appendicitis is made on the basis of the history and physical exam.

Choose the **BEST** response.

389.   If pain fibers in the inflamed appendix produce visceral pain, in which abdominal region or regions will the patient **MOST** likely feel the visceral pain?

     (A)   epigastric and/or umbilical
     (B)   hypogastric
     (C)   right hypochondriac
     (D)   right lumbar
     (E)   right inguinal

390. Assume that the appendix in the patient lies anterior to the terminal ileum, and that inflammation of the appendix has extended to the anterolateral abdominal wall in contact with the appendix. Physical examination of the patient as this time is likely to show all of the following findings **EXCEPT**:

   (A)   Deep tenderness in the right lower quadrant (RLQ) upon deep palpation of the RLQ.
   (B)   Deep tenderness in the RLQ upon deep palpation of the left lower quadrant (LLQ).
   (C)   Pain in the abdominal wall of the RLQ when fingers are pressed into the abdominal wall of the RLQ and then suddenly withdrawn.
   (D)   Pain in the abdominal wall of the RLQ when fingers are pressed into the abdominal wall of the LLQ and then suddenly withdrawn.
   (E)   Right-sided rectal tenderness when right-sided pressure is applied to the rectum during a rectal exam.

391. Assume that the appendix in the patient lies directly posterior to the cecum, and that inflammation of the appendix has extended to the posterior abdominal wall in contact with the appendix. Physical examination of the patient as this time is **MOST** likely to show pain upon

   (A)   abduction of the right thigh against resistance
   (B)   flexion of the right thigh against resistance
   (C)   adduction of the right thigh against resistance
   (D)   passive internal rotation of the right thigh
   (E)   passive external rotation of the left thigh

ANSWERS AND TUTORIAL ON ITEMS 389-391

The answers are: **389-A; 390-E; 391-B**. Disease or injury of the abdominal viscera supplied by the **superior mesenteric artery** (which include the appendix) produces visceral **pain** that is most commonly localized to the **umbilical region**. However, an inflamed appendix may elicit painful, contractive spasm of the pyloric sphincter. Stimulation of visceral pain fibers in the abdominal viscera supplied by the celiac artery (which include the pyloric region of the stomach) produces visceral pain that is most commonly localized to the epigastric region. Accordingly, appendicitis may produce visceral pain localized to the epigastric and/or umbilical regions.

Localized **deep tenderness in the RLQ** is a common symptom of **appendicitis** prior to perforation. The deep tenderness is either wholly or in part visceral pain that emanates from the appendix upon the application of external pressure, and thus the site of deep tenderness always corresponds to the location of the appendix. Deep palpation of either the RLQ or LLQ may produce sufficient external pressure upon the inflamed appendix to elicit deep tenderness in the

RLQ, particularly if the appendix lies within the right lateral paracolic gutter (alongside the cecum) (position A in **Figure 3.49**), on the parietal peritoneum overlying the iliacus muscle in the iliac fossa (position B), or anterior to the terminal ileum (position C). If the appendix lies posterior to the cecum (position D) or draped over the right lateral wall of the pelvis (position E), deep palpation of the lower quadrants may not produce sufficient external pressure upon the inflamed appendix to elicit deep tenderness in the RLQ.

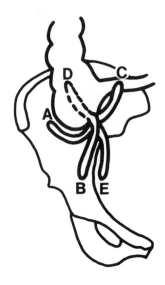

Figure 3.49

Inflamed parietal peritoneum is exquisitely sensitive to sudden changes in tension. Such sensitivity in the parietal peritoneum of the anterolateral abdominal wall can be detected by an examiner pressing the approximated fingers of one hand deep into a region of the patient's anterolateral abdominal wall and then suddenly withdrawing the fingers. The wave of sudden rebound movement which spreads throughout the abdominal walls elicits tenderness in those wall regions lined by inflamed parietal peritoneum. It is preferable to apply the finger pressure at a site distant from the suspected sites of inflammation. The examiner must use discretion in applying appropriate pressure during testing for **rebound tenderness**, as the pain can be quite severe.

When an inflamed appendix lies in position B or D, its inflammatory process can readily extend posteriorly to the iliacus muscle in the right iliac fossa. Right iliopsoas inflammation is indicated if there is pain upon active flexion of the right thigh against resistance or pain upon passive hyperextension of the right thigh.

When an inflamed appendix lies in position E, its inflammatory process can readily extend laterally to the obturator internus muscle in the right lateral pelvic wall or medially to the right side of the rectum. Right obturator internus inflammation is indicated if there is pain upon passive external and internal rotation of the right thigh, and right-sided rectal inflammation is indicated if there is right-sided rectal tenderness upon rectal exam.

Items 392-394

The following items concern visceral pain associated with disease of the large intestine and the blood supply and parasympathetic innervation of the large intestine.

Choose the **BEST** response.

392. If a diverticulum of the sigmoid colon became inflamed, in which abdominal region will the individual **MOST** likely feel the visceral pain?

    (A)   left inguinal region
    (B)   left lumbar region
    (C)   epigastric region
    (D)   umbilical region
    (E)   hypogastric region

393. Where along the course of the large intestine do colic branches of the superior mesenteric artery anastomose with colic branches of the inferior mesenteric artery?

    (A)   near the border between the cecum and ascending colon
    (B)   near the hepatic flexure
    (C)   near the splenic flexure
    (D)   near the border between the descending colon and sigmoid colon
    (E)   near the border between the sigmoid colon and rectum

394. The vagus nerves provide preganglionic parasympathetic innervation to the large intestine as far distally as the region near the

    (A)   border between the cecum and ascending colon
    (B)   hepatic flexure
    (C)   splenic flexure
    (D)   border between the descending colon and sigmoid colon
    (E)   border between the sigmoid colon and rectum

ANSWERS AND TUTORIAL ON ITEMS 392-394

The answers are: **392-E; 393-C; 394-C**. Disease or injury of the abdominal viscera supplied by the **inferior mesenteric artery** (which include the sigmoid colon) produces visceral pain that is most commonly localized to the **hypogastric region**. The terminal branches of the ileocolic (IC), right colic (RC), and middle colic (MC) branches of the superior mesenteric artery extend distally along the large intestine as far the border region between the middle and left thirds of

199

the transverse colon (**Figure 3.50**). The terminal branches of the left colic (LC) and sigmoid (S) branches of the inferior mesenteric artery extend along the distal third of the transverse colon and the entire lengths of the descending and sigmoid colons. The anastomoses among the terminal branches of the colic branches of the superior and inferior mesenteric arteries form, in effect, an artery that runs along the medial margins of the ascending and descending colons and the mesenteric margins of the transverse and sigmoid colons. This artery is called the **marginal artery of Drummond**.

The **vagus nerves** provide preganglionic parasympathetic innervation along the large intestine as far distally as the border region between the middle and left thirds of the transverse colon. The pelvic splanchnic nerves provide preganglionic parasympathetic innervation to the remaining distal segments of the large intestine.

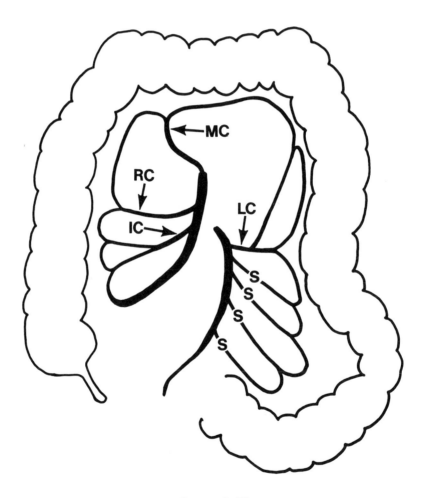

Figure 3.50

Items 395-402

A 31-year-old man complains of excruciating abdominal pain during the last 2 hours. A tentative diagnosis of ureteral obstruction is made on the basis of the history and physical exam. An intravenous urogram showing obstruction of the right ureter by a radiodense calculus at the ureteropelvic junction confirms the diagnosis.

Choose the **BEST** response.

395. The pain of ureteral colic may involve all of the following regions **EXCEPT**:

    (A)   ipsilateral shoulder
    (B)   ipsilateral costovertebral region
    (C)   ipsilateral lumbar, or flank, region
    (D)   ipsilateral inguinal region
    (E)   ipsilateral scrotum or vulva

396. Sensory fibers from the upper part of the ureter enter the spinal cord at spinal cord segment levels

    (A)   T1, T2, T3, T4, and T5
    (B)   T5, T6, T7, T8, and T9
    (C)   T8, T9, T10, T11, and T12
    (D)   T10, T11, T12, L1, and L2
    (E)   L1, L2, S2, S3, and S4

397. An individual suffering from acute pyelonephritis commonly exhibits tenderness upon gentle fist percussion of the back region overlying the inflamed kidney. The gentle fist percussion is applied immediately lateral to the vertebral column at the level of the

    (A)   6th thoracic vertebra
    (B)   8th thoracic vertebra
    (C)   10th thoracic vertebra
    (D)   12th thoracic vertebra
    (E)   4th lumbar vertebra

398. The length of an adult kidney (the distance between its superior and inferior poles) averages _____ times the thickness of the body of the 2nd lumbar vertebra.

    (A)   1.5
    (B)   2.6
    (C)   3.7
    (D)   4.8
    (E)   5.9

399. All of the following statements concerning the blood supply and venous drainage of the adrenal glands are correct **EXCEPT**:

(A) Both are supplied by direct branches of the inferior phrenic artery.
(B) Both are supplied by direct branches of the abdominal aorta.
(C) Both are supplied by direct branches of the renal artery.
(D) The left adrenal vein commonly ends by union with the inferior vena cava.
(E) The right adrenal vein commonly ends by union with the inferior vena cava.

In the following items, match each part of the kidney with its representation in **Figure 3.51** below, a drawing of a coronally-sectioned kidney.

400. Renal pyramid

401. Renal column

402. Minor calyx

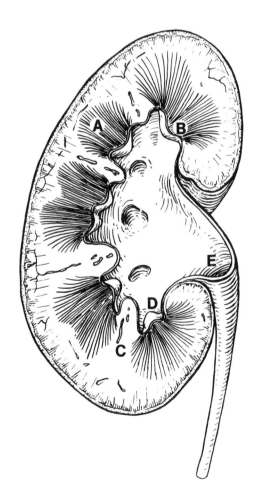

Figure 3.51

ANSWERS AND TUTORIAL ON ITEMS 395-402

The answers are: **395-A; 396-D; 397-D; 398-C; 399-D; 400-A; 401-C; 402-D. Intravenous urograms** permit evaluation of kidney position, size, and parenchymal thickness; the shape of the renal papillae and calyces; and the presence of filling defects in calyces and/or ureter.

Disease or injury of the upper part of the **ureter** produces visceral pain that is frequently localized to the **costovertebral region**. Disease or injury of the upper part of the ureter may refer pain to parts of the T10-L2 dermatomes, which include the flank and inguinal regions of the abdomen and the scrotum or vulva.

Disease or injury of the **kidney** produces visceral pain that is most commonly localized to the **costovertebral region**. Deep tenderness upon gentle fist percussion to the costovertebral region (CVR) (the back region immediately inferior to the posterior part of the 12th rib and immediately lateral to the bodies of the 12th thoracic and 1st lumbar vertebrae) suggests kidney disease or injury (**Figure 3.52**).

The envelope of perirenal fat occasionally permits visualization of the superior and inferior poles of a kidney in an abdominal plain film. Comparison of the length of the kidney relative to the thickness of the body of the 2nd lumbar vertebra can be used to assess if the kidney is within normal size limits. The left adrenal vein commonly ends by union with the left renal vein. In the drawing of the coronally sectioned view of the kidney, the part labelled B is a renal papilla, and the part labelled E is the pelvis of the ureter.

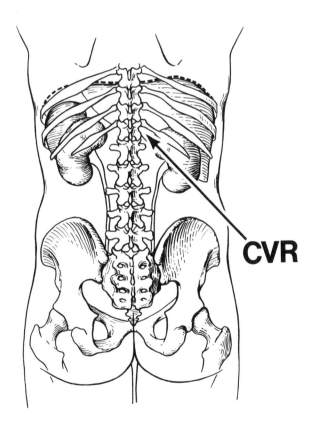

Figure 3.52

The following items address information relevant to disease and disorders of pelvic and perineal viscera.

Choose the **BEST** response.

403. Which of the following structures **MOST** strongly supports the uterus in the pelvis?

    (A) broad ligament of the uterus
    (B) levator ani
    (C) transverse cervical ligament
    (D) round ligament of the uterus
    (E) uterosacral ligament

404. **MOST** of the lymph collected from the fundus of the uterus drains into the

    (A) aortic nodes
    (B) external iliac nodes
    (C) internal iliac nodes
    (D) horizontal group of superficial inguinal nodes
    (E) vertical group of superficial inguinal nodes

405. **MOST** of the lymph collected from the lower half of the anal canal drains into the

    (A) aortic nodes
    (B) external iliac nodes
    (C) internal iliac nodes
    (D) horizontal group of superficial inguinal nodes
    (E) vertical group of superficial inguinal nodes

406. All of the following statements concerning digital examination of the anal canal and rectum are correct **EXCEPT**:

    (A) The intermuscular groove marks the lower border of the internal anal sphincter.
    (B) The anorectal ring marks the upper border of the external anal sphincter.
    (C) In a male, the prostate can be palpated through the anterior wall of the rectum.
    (D) In a female, the cervix of the uterus can generally be palpated through the anterior wall of the rectum.
    (E) In a female, the fundus of an anteverted and anteflexed uterus can generally be palpated through the anterior wall of the rectum.

407. All of the following statements concerning penile erection and ejaculation are correct **EXCEPT**:

   (A)   Terminal branches of the internal pudendal arteries supply of the erectile tissues of the penis.
   (B)   Increased sympathetic activity during sexual arousal increases blood flow to the erectile tissues of the penis.
   (C)   Penile erection occurs as a consequence of the engorgement of the cavernous sinuses in the corpora cavernosa of the penis.
   (D)   Secretions from the seminal vesicles and prostate gland contribute to the ejaculate.
   (E)   Ejaculation occurs as a consequence of the rhythmic contractions of the bulbospongiosus muscles.

408. All of the following statements concerning the bladder are correct **EXCEPT**:

   (A)   Disease or injury of the bladder produces visceral pain that is most commonly localized to the suprapubic region.
   (B)   Disease or injury of the bladder may refer pain to parts of the L1, L2, S2, S3, and S4 dermatomes.
   (C)   Micturition requires voluntary relaxation of the sphincter urethrae.
   (D)   Contraction of the anterolateral abdominal wall musculature and the diaphragm can aid micturition.
   (E)   Micturition requires voluntary contraction of the levator ani.

ANSWERS AND TUTORIAL ON ITEMS 403-408

The answers are: **403-B; 404-A; 405-D; 406-E; 407-B; 408-E**. The principal supports of the **uterus** are the paired **levator ani muscles**. Two paired condensations of endopelvic fascia attached to the cervix of the uterus and vault of the vagina (the cardinal, or transverse cervical, ligaments and the uterosacral ligaments) provide **secondary support**. The cardinal ligaments extend from the lateral pelvic walls to the cervix and vagina along the lowest margin of the extraperitoneal space within the broad ligaments of the uterus; the cardinal ligaments help stabilize the midline position of the cervix and the vault of the vagina. The uterosacral ligaments arise from the lower end of the sacrum and extend anteriorly around the sides of the rectum to attach to the cervix and vagina; the uterosacral ligaments securely tether the cervix to the sacrum, and help stabilize the approximately 90° angle between the longitudinal axes of the vagina (V) and the cervix of the uterus (CU) (**Figure 3.53**).

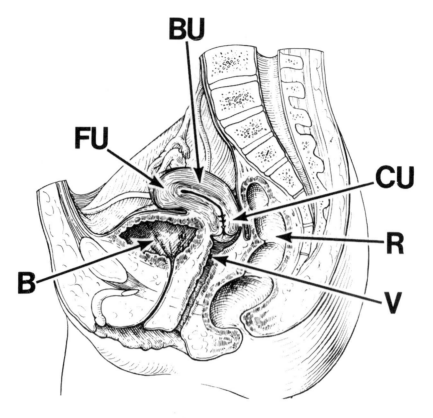

Figure 3.53

Lymph collected from the lower third of the vagina drains into the horizontal group of **superficial inguinal nodes**. Lymph collected from the middle third of the vagina drains into internal iliac nodes. Lymph collected from the upper third of the vagina drains into external and internal iliac nodes. Most of the lymph collected from the cervix and body of the uterus drains into internal iliac nodes. Lymph collected from the fundus of the uterus, the uterine tubes, and the ovaries drains into aortic nodes at the level of the body of the 1st lumbar vertebra.

Lymph collected from the upper half of the anal canal and the lower half of the rectum drains into internal iliac nodes. Lymph collected from the upper half of the rectum drains into the inferior mesenteric nodes.

When the urinary bladder (B) is empty, it is common for the uterus to be both anteverted and anteflexed (**Figure 3.53**). An anteverted uterus has its longitudinal axis bent forward (generally at an approximately 90° angle) relative to the longitudinal axis of the vagina (V). An anteflexed uterus has its body (BU) bent forward relative to the cervix (CU). The cervix of the uterus can generally be palpated through the anterior wall of the rectum (R). The fundus (FU) of an anteverted and anteflexed uterus may be palpated during bimanual examination of the pelvis.

In the male, the **prostate** (P) can be palpated through the anterior wall of the rectum (R) (**Figure 3.54**).

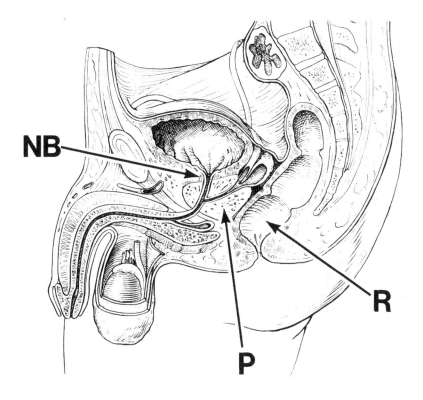

Figure 3.54

Increased parasympathetic activity during sexual arousal increases blood flow to the erectile tissues of the penis.

The act of **micturition** requires voluntary relaxation of the paired levator ani muscles and the sphincter urethrae. The relaxation of the levator ani not only pulls the neck of the bladder (NB) downward (and thus decreasing the resistance in the neck), but also reflexively stimulates contraction of the detrusor (**Figure 3.54**). The detrusor is the smooth muscle tissue in the bladder wall; it is innervated by parasympathetic fibers provided via the pelvic splanchnic nerves.

The five CT scans in **Figure 3.55** are adjacent 10 mm-thick scans of the upper abdomen. The radiopacity of the blood vessels has been enhanced by intravenously injected contrast material. In the following items, match each structure with its image in the labelled CT scans.

409.   Caudate lobe of liver

410.   Splenic vein

411.   Inferior vena cava

412.   Portal vein

413.   Body of pancreas

414.   Left adrenal gland

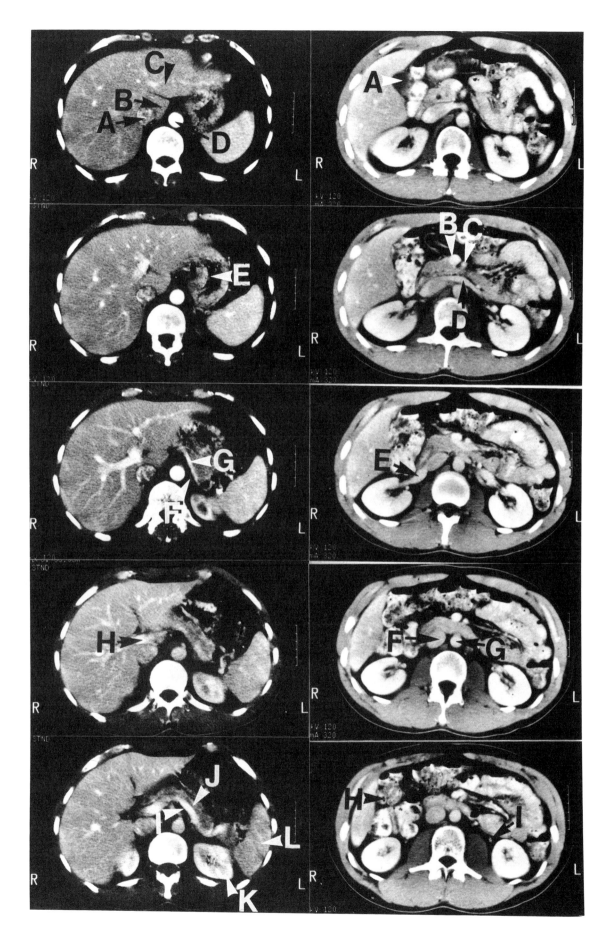

Figure 3.55　　　　　　　　**Figure 3.56**

The answers are: **409-B; 410-I; 411-A; 412-H; 413-J; 414-F**. C is the left lobe of the liver. D is the abdominal aorta. E is body of the stomach. G is the splenic artery. K is the left kidney. L is the spleen.

Figure 3.55 shows (i) the body of the stomach lying posterior to the left lobe of the liver and (ii) the spleen suspended in the posterolateral aspect of the left upper quadrant of the abdomen. The caudate lobe of the liver is shown bordered between the inferior vena cava and the fissure extending into the visceral surface of the liver. The third scan shows the splenic artery following a serpentine course to the hilum of the spleen. The arrowhead-shaped structure lying immediately anteromedial to the upper pole of the left kidney represents the left adrenal gland. The highlighted vessels in the liver represent divisions of the portal vein. The fourth scan shows the portal vein entering the liver via the porta hepatis. The fifth scan shows that as the splenic vein extends rightward from the hilum of the spleen, it passes posterior to the body of the pancreas. In distinguishing the splenic artery from the splenic vein in CT scans of the upper abdomen, observe that whereas the splenic artery is best visualized at levels above that of the body of the pancreas (such as the level shown in the third scan), the splenic vein is identified by its posterior relationship to the body of the pancreas.

Items 415-418

The five CT scans in **Figure 3.56** are adjacent 10 mm-thick scans of the mid abdomen. In the following items, match each structure with its image in the labelled CT scans.

415.   Left renal vein

416.   Superior mesenteric artery

417.   Abdominal aorta

418.   Left ureter

ANSWERS AND TUTORIAL ON ITEMS 415-418

The answers are: **415-D; 416-C; 417-G; 418-I**. A is the fundus of the gallbladder. B is the superior mesenteric vein. E is the right renal vein. F is the inferior vena cava. H is the ascending colon. The first scan shows the fundus of the gallbladder pressed into the visceral surface of the liver on its right. The cross sectional area occupied by the liver progressively decreases as we proceed from the first to the fifth scan. The second scan shows the left renal vein crossing anterior to the abdominal aorta in route to its union with the inferior vena cava. The superior mesenteric artery and superior mesenteric vein lie anterior to the duodenum; the superior mesenteric artery lies to the left of the vein and has a smaller cross-sectional area than the vein. The third scan shows the union of the right renal vein with the inferior vena cava. The right renal vein lies at a level lower than that of the left renal vein because the right kidney typically rests at a level lower than that of the left kidney. The fourth scan shows the abdominal aorta anterior to and slightly to the left of a lumbar vertebra and the inferior vena cava anterior to and slightly to the right of the lumbar vertebra. The fifth scan shows the descending colon to the left of the liver. The left ureter lies immediately anterolateral to the left psoas major muscle.

Items 419-420

A 23-year-old man hit his head when he fell from his bicycle. His cycling helmet protected him against skull fractures but did not prevent him from becoming permanently anosmic as a result of tearing of the first-order nerve fibers of both olfactory nerves.

Choose the **BEST** response.

419. Which part of the ethmoid bone transmits the nerve fibers of the olfactory nerve from the nasal cavity to the cranial cavity?

   (A)   perpendicular plate
   (B)   cribriform plate
   (C)   superior concha
   (D)   middle concha
   (E)   crista galli

420. The ethmoid bone contributes to the bony foundation of all of the following **EXCEPT**:

(A)   roof of the nasal cavity
(B)   lateral wall of the nasal cavity
(C)   nasal septum
(D)   floor of the nasal cavity
(E)   medial wall of the orbital cavity

ANSWERS AND TUTORIAL ON ITEMS 419-420

The answers are: **419-B; 420-D.** The **olfactory nerve** (cranial nerve I) arises from first-order sensory neurons which lie within the mucosal lining of the roof of the nasal cavity. The afferent fibers of these first-order neurons extend from the nasal cavity into the cranial cavity by passing through perforations in the cribriform plate of the ethmoid bone. These fibers extend into the olfactory bulb to synapse with second-order neurons. Afferent fibers of the second-order neurons extend posteriorly through the olfactory tract to enter the brain. Blows to the head which displace the brain posteriorly can produce tears in the afferent fibers of the first-order neurons of the olfactory nerve near the sites where the fibers emerge from the perforations in the cribriform plate of the ethmoid bone.

The **cribriform plate** of the ethmoid bone forms the bony foundation of the roof of the nasal cavity. The perpendicular plate of the ethmoid bone forms part of the bony foundation of the nasal septum. The superior and middle conchae form part of the bony foundation of the lateral wall of the nasal cavity. The orbital plate of the ethmoid bone forms part of the bony foundation of the medial wall of the orbital cavity. The palatine process of the maxillary bone and the horizontal plate of the palatine bone form the bony foundation of the floor of the nasal cavity.

Invasive tumors of the sphenoid bone may press upon and impair the nerves that extend through the superior orbital fissure.

Choose the **BEST** response.

421. All of the following nerves extend through the superior orbital fissure **EXCEPT:**

   (A) ophthalmic division of the trigeminal nerve
   (B) oculomotor nerve
   (C) optic nerve
   (D) trochlear nerve
   (E) abducent nerve

422. All of the following movements could be weakened or lost as a result of injury to the nerves that extend through the superior orbital fissure **EXCEPT:**

   (A) directing the pupil laterally
   (B) directing the pupil medially
   (C) forcibly closing the eyelids
   (D) raising the upper eyelid
   (E) pupillary constriction

423. All of the following regions could loose the sense of touch by injury to nerves extending through the superior orbital fissure **EXCEPT:**

   (A) forehead
   (B) tip of the nose
   (C) cornea
   (D) upper eyelid
   (E) lower eyelid

The answers are: **421-C; 422-C; 423-E.** The superior orbital fissure is a slit between the greater and lesser wings of the **sphenoid bone**. It transmits the oculomotor nerve, trochlear nerve, ophthalmic division of the trigeminal nerve and abducent nerve between the cranial and orbital cavities.

The **optic nerve** (cranial nerve II) extends from the orbital to the cranial cavity by passing through the optic canal, a passageway that traverses the body and lesser wing of the sphenoid bone.

The **oculomotor nerve** (cranial nerve III) innervates four of the extraocular muscles of the eyeball (medial rectus, superior rectus, inferior rectus and inferior oblique) and levator palpebrae superioris. Medial rectus moves the eyeball medially. Levator palpebrae superioris raises the upper eyelid. The oculomotor nerve also transmits preganglionic parasympathetic fibers which synapse with postganglionic parasympathetic neurons in the ciliary ganglion. The ciliary ganglion lies in the orbital cavity posterior to the eyeball. The postganglionic parasympathetic fibers which emanate from the ciliary ganglion innervate two intraocular muscles: sphincter pupillae (which acts to decrease the size of the pupil) and ciliaris (which acts to focus the lens on near objects).

The trochlear nerve (cranial nerve IV) innervates the extraocular muscle superior oblique. The ophthalmic division of the trigeminal nerve (cranial nerve V) provides sensory innervation for (a) the mucous membrane lining the anterior third of the nasal cavity, frontal sinus, sphenoid sinus and part of the ethmoid air cells, (b) the bulbar conjunctiva of the eyeball and the palpebral conjunctiva of the upper eyelid and (c) the skin of the forehead, the upper eyelid and the bridge and tip of the nose. The maxillary division of the trigeminal nerve provides sensory innervation for the skin of the lower eyelid.

The abducent nerve (cranial nerve VI) innervates lateral rectus. When acting alone, lateral rectus moves the eyeball laterally. The facial nerve (cranial nerve VII) innervates orbicularis oculi (OO), the muscle of facial expression responsible for forcibly closing the eyelids (**Figure 3.57**).

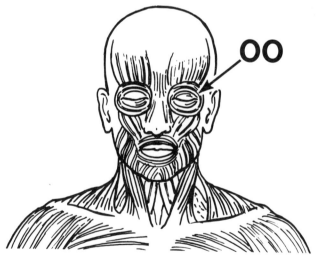

Figure 3.57

214

Items 424-426

A 38-year-old woman with septic thrombosis of the cavernous sinus complains of double vision whenever she looks downward. The two images are farthest apart when she looks downward and to the left. The physical exam shows that the patient can move her right eyeball directly to the left. However, when her right eyeball faces directly medially, the patient is unable to move her right eyeball downward.

424.   Which muscle of her right eye is **NOT** acting effectively?

    (A)   superior rectus
    (B)   inferior rectus
    (C)   lateral rectus
    (D)   inferior oblique
    (E)   superior oblique

425.   All of the following structures extend through the interior of the cavernous sinus or its lateral wall **EXCEPT:**

    (A)   postganglionic sympathetic fibers that innervate dilator pupillae
    (B)   internal carotid artery
    (C)   trochlear nerve
    (D)   maxillary division of the trigeminal nerve
    (E)   mandibular division of the trigeminal nerve

426.   All of the following statements concerning the cavernous sinus are correct **EXCEPT:**

    (A)   The cavernous sinus lies immediately lateral the pituitary gland.
    (B)   The cavernous sinus lies immediately medial to the frontal lobe of the cerebrum.
    (C)   The cavernous sinus can drain blood from the facial vein.
    (D)   The superior ophthalmic vein is a tributary of the cavernous sinus.
    (E)   The internal jugular vein can drain blood from the cavernous sinus.

ANSWERS AND TUTORIAL ON ITEMS 424-426

The answers are: **424-E; 425-E; 426-B.** The **cavernous sinus** lies medial to the temporal lobe of the cerebral hemisphere. **Septic thrombosis** of the cavernous sinus may inflame and injure the nerves that extend through the interior of the sinus or its lateral wall. The lateral wall of the cavernous sinus transmits segments of the oculomotor nerve, the ophthalmic and maxillary divisions of the trigeminal nerve and the trochlear nerve. The interior of the cavernous sinus is traversed by segments of the abducent nerve and the internal carotid artery (and accompanying postganglionic sympathetic fibers, some of which innervate dilator pupillae).

The **medial** and **lateral rectus muscles** move the eyeball from its primary position to orientations in which the cornea faces, respectively, directly medially and laterally. The activities of the medial and lateral rectus muscles are tested during a physical exam by asking the patient to look in directions that directly match the actions of these muscles. For example, to test the activity of the medial rectus, the patient is asked to try to look at the nose. In this case involving a patient with diplopia, the medial rectus of the right eye functions normally.

The **superior** and **inferior rectus muscles** move the eyeball from its primary position to orientations in which the cornea faces, respectively, superomedially and inferomedially. The superior and inferior oblique muscles move the eyeball from its primary position to orientations in which the cornea faces, respectively, inferolaterally and superolaterally. However, in testing the activities of the superior and inferior recti and the superior and inferior obliques, the patient is asked to look in directions that do not correspond to the actions of these muscles. With the cornea facing directly laterally (that is, with the patient looking directly to the side of the head), the activities of the superior and inferior rectus muscles are tested by asking the patient to look, respectively, upward and downward. With the cornea facing directly medially (that is, with the patient looking directly at the nose), the activities of the superior and inferior obliques are tested by asking the patient to look, respectively, downward and upward. **Figure 3.58** is a drawing of the superior view of the relationship of the superior oblique muscle (SO) to the right eyeball. Notice that if the cornea (C) faces directly medially, superior oblique is the only extraocular muscle whose actions can move the eyeball so that the cornea also faces inferiorly.

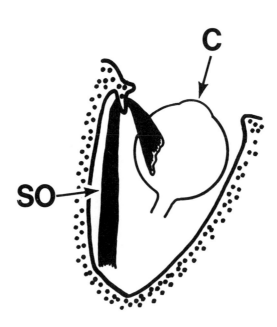

Figure 3.58

Items 427-430

The following items pertain to tests that can be performed to examine cranial nerve function.

Choose the **BEST** response.

427. The jaw jerk is a deep tendon reflex in which tapping a patient's lower jaw causes a reflexive raising of the lower jaw. The jaw jerk tests sensory fibers of the

    (A) mandibular division of the trigeminal nerve
    (B) facial nerve
    (C) glossopharyngeal nerve
    (D) vagus nerve and cranial root of the accessory nerve
    (E) hypoglossal nerve

428. The jaw jerk tests motor fibers of the

    (A) mandibular division of the trigeminal nerve
    (B) facial nerve
    (C) glossopharyngeal nerve
    (D) vagus nerve and cranial root of the accessory nerve
    (E) hypoglossal nerve

429. Palpation of the masseter muscle as the patient is asked to clench the teeth tests motor fibers of the

    (A) mandibular division of the trigeminal nerve
    (B) facial nerve
    (C) glossopharyngeal nerve
    (D) vagus nerve and cranial root of the accessory nerve
    (E) hypoglossal nerve

430. During mirror laryngoscopy, an examiner notes paralysis of the right vocal fold (the right vocal fold is not abducted when the patient is requested to say "e-e-e" in a high-pitched voice). This indicates paralysis of muscles innervated by the

    (A) mandibular division of the trigeminal nerve
    (B) facial nerve
    (C) glossopharyngeal nerve
    (D) vagus nerve and cranial root of the accessory nerve
    (E) hypoglossal nerve

ANSWERS AND TUTORIAL ON ITEMS 427-430

The answers are: **427-A; 428-A; 429-A; 430-D.** The stretch receptors and muscle fibers of the **muscles of mastication** (temporalis, masseter, lateral pterygoid and medial pterygoid) are innervated by the mandibular division of the **trigeminal nerve**. Masseter and medial pterygoid raise the lower jaw at the **temporomandibular joint** (TMJ). The tone of the masseters increases when an individual clenches the teeth. Temporalis raises and retracts the lower jaw at the TMJ. Lateral pterygoid lowers and protracts the lower jaw.

The **intrinsic muscles of the larynx** (which are the muscles that abduct, adduct, tense and relax the vocal folds) are innervated by branches of the vagus nerves. Almost all of the motor nerve fibers to the intrinsic muscles of the larynx are from the cranial root of the accessory nerve (which joins the vagus nerve in the uppermost part of the neck). With the exception of the cricothyroids, all the intrinsic muscles of the larynx are innervated by the recurrent laryngeal nerves. The cricothyroids are innervated by the external laryngeal nerves. The muscles chiefly responsible for abducting the vocal folds during **phonation** are the **posterior cricoarytenoid muscles**.

Items 431-437

The following items pertain to tests that can be performed to examine cranial nerve function.

Choose the **BEST** response.

431. A patient is asked to stick out her tongue and a left deviation is noted. If this problem is a result of disease or injury to motor nerve fibers, then it **MOST** likely indicates injury to the

    (A)   mandibular division of the left trigeminal nerve
    (B)   left vagus nerve and cranial root of the left accessory nerve
    (C)   right vagus nerve and cranial root of the right accessory nerve
    (D)   left hypoglossal nerve
    (E)   right hypoglossal nerve

432. A patient is asked to stick out her tongue and say "ahhhh" and left deviation of the uvula and soft palate is noted. If this problem is a result of disease or injury to motor nerve fibers, then it **MOST** likely indicates injury to the

    (A)   left glossopharyngeal nerve
    (B)   left vagus nerve and cranial root of the left accessory nerve
    (C)   right vagus nerve and cranial root of the right accessory nerve
    (D)   left hypoglossal nerve
    (E)   right hypoglossal nerve

433. A patient is asked to smile and it is noted that the left corner of her mouth does not move upward. If this problem is a result of disease or injury to motor nerve fibers, then it **MOST** likely indicates injury to the

   (A)   mandibular division of the left trigeminal nerve
   (B)   left facial nerve
   (C)   left glossopharyngeal nerve
   (D)   left vagus nerve and cranial root of the left accessory nerve
   (E)   left hypoglossal nerve

434. An examiner massages a patient's neck in the region overlying the carotid pulse and notes a reflexive decrease in the rate of the patient's heartbeat. This reflex slowing of the heart is mediated by preganglionic parasympathetic fibers of the

   (A)   facial nerve
   (B)   glossopharyngeal nerve
   (C)   vagus nerve
   (D)   cranial root of the accessory nerve
   (E)   hypoglossal nerve

435. The nerve that is the origin for taste fibers on the tip of the tongue is the

   (A)   mandibular division of the trigeminal nerve
   (B)   facial nerve
   (C)   glossopharyngeal nerve
   (D)   vagus nerve
   (E)   hypoglossal nerve

436. The nerve that provide sensation for light touch on the tip of the tongue is/are the

   (A)   mandibular division of the trigeminal nerve
   (B)   facial nerve
   (C)   glossopharyngeal nerve
   (D)   vagus nerve
   (E)   hypoglossal nerve

437. The muscle **MOST** responsible for protrusion of the tongue is the

   (A)   intrinsic muscles of the tongue
   (B)   palatoglossus
   (C)   genioglossus
   (D)   styloglossus
   (E)   hyoglossus

The answers are: **431-D; 432-C; 433-B; 434-C; 435-B; 436-A; 437-C.** Genioglossus, hyoglossus, styloglossus and all the intrinsic muscles of the tongue are innervated by the **hypoglossal nerve. Genioglossus** is the only extrinsic muscle of the tongue which can protrude the tongue. When genioglossus acts to protrude the tip of the tongue, it also deviates the tip of the tongue to the contralateral side. Consequently, denervation of the left genioglossus will cause left lingual deviation, since the left genioglossus cannot oppose the leftward thrust of the right genioglossus.

Musculus uvula and levator veli palatini raise and pull the uvula to the ipsilateral side. Denervation the left musculus uvula and levator veli palatini will cause the uvula to deviate to the right when the individual says "ah," since the left musculus uvula and levator veli palatini cannot oppose the rightward pull of the right musculus uvula and levator veli palatini. Almost all of the motor nerve fibers to musculus uvula and levator veli palatini are from the cranial root of the accessory nerve (which joins the vagus nerve in the uppermost part of the neck). The muscles of facial expression are responsible for the appearance of a smile, and are innervated by the terminal branches of the facial nerve.

The origin of the internal carotid artery exhibits a dilatation called the **carotid sinus** (the carotid sinus may also be located at the termination of the common carotid artery). Each carotid sinus bears many baroreceptors innervated chiefly by the glossopharyngeal nerve. When these fibers are subjected to a sudden change in blood pressure, their response initiates an autonomic reflex which restores the blood pressure back to normal levels. The restoration occurs via regulation of arteriolar constriction and heart rate. A sudden increase in blood pressure stimulates the parasympathetic innervation of the cardiac plexuses by the vagus nerves. The parasympathetic stimulation decreases the heart rate.

The chorda tympani branch of the **facial nerve** provides taste sensation for the anterior two-thirds of the tongue. The mandibular division of the trigeminal nerve provides sensory innervation for the anterior two-thirds of the tongue. The glossopharyngeal nerve provides both sensory innervation and taste sensation for the posterior third of the tongue.

The functions served by the **facial nerve** include the following:

[1]   Its greater petrosal branch provides preganglionic parasympathetic innervation for the lacrimal gland and the mucosal glands of the nasal cavity. The preganglionic parasympathetic fibers synapse with postganglionic parasympathetic neurons in the pterygopalatine ganglion.

[2]   It innervates stapedius, a muscle of the middle ear.

[3]   Its chorda tympani branch provides taste sensation for the anterior two-thirds of the tongue and preganglionic parasympathetic innervation for the submandibular and sublingual salivary glands. The preganglionic parasympathetic fibers synapse with postganglionic parasympathetic neurons in the submandibular ganglion.

[4]   Its terminal branches innervate stylohyoid, the posterior belly of digastric and all the muscles of facial expression.

The functions served by the **glossopharyngeal nerve** include the following:

[1]   Its lesser petrosal branch provides preganglionic parasympathetic innervation for the parotid salivary gland. The preganglionic parasympathetic fibers synapse with postganglionic parasympathetic neurons in the otic ganglion.

[2]   It innervates stylopharyngeus.

[3]   It provides sensory innervation for the posterior third of the tongue, the lower half of the nasopharynx and all of the oropharynx and laryngopharynx. The vagus nerve also provides sensory innervation for the oropharynx and laryngopharynx.

[4]   It provides taste sensation for the posterior third of the tongue.

[5]   It supplies the baroreceptors of the carotid sinus.

[6]   It supplies the chemoreceptors of the carotid body.

Items 438-440

The two CT scans in **Figure 3.59** are adjacent 10 mm-thick scans of the head. Contrast material was administered intravenously prior to the scans. Match each item with its image in the labeled CT scan.

438.   Mastoid air cells

439.   Sphenoid sinuses

440.   External auditory meatus

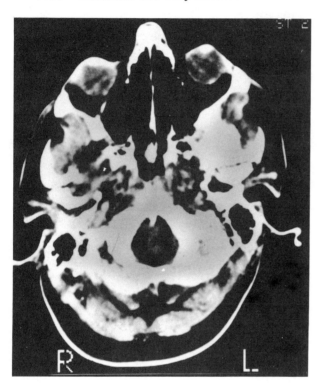 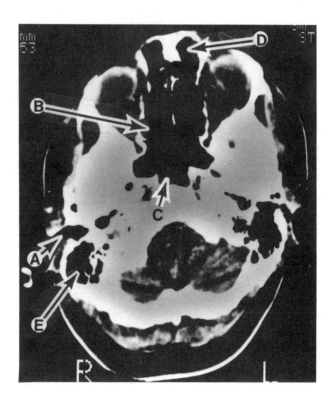

Figure 3.59

ANSWERS AND TUTORIAL ON ITEMS 438-440

The answers are: **438-E; 439-C; 440-A.** CT images such as those shown in **Figure 3.59** depict bone as intense white and air, fluid and other tissues as gray to black. A is the right external acoustic meatus. B marks the right ethmoid air cells. C indicates the sphenoid sinus. D is the left frontal sinus. E indicates the right mastoid air cells.

CHAPTER IV
NEUROANATOMY

Items 441-445

Figure 4.1 is a cross-section through the brainstem.

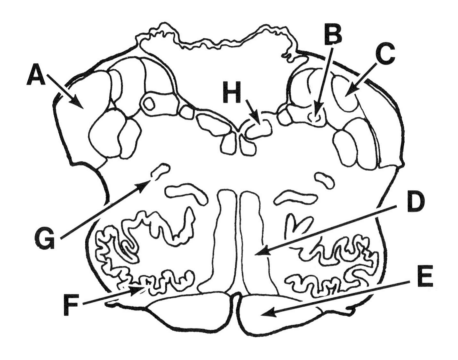

Figure 4.1

Choose the **BEST** response.

441.   The cross-section represents what portion of the brainstem?

   (A)   rostral pons
   (B)   midbrain
   (C)   rostral medulla
   (D)   caudal medulla
   (E)   caudal pons

442. Which labeled structure carries proprioceptive information from the limbs?

    (A)   A
    (B)   B
    (C)   C
    (D)   D
    (E)   E

443.   The origin of most of the axons found in structure E is the

    (A)   cerebellum
    (B)   motor and premotor cortex
    (C)   spinal cord
    (D)   caudate nucleus
    (E)   red nucleus

444.   Which structure provides motor innervation to the muscles of the soft palate and pharynx?

    (A)   D
    (B)   E
    (C)   F
    (D)   G
    (E)   H

445.   The portion of the ventricular system found at this level of the brainstem is the

    (A)   open portion of the 4th ventricle
    (B)   cerebral aqueduct
    (C)   3rd ventricle
    (D)   central canal
    (E)   lateral ventricle

ANSWERS AND TUTORIAL ON ITEMS 441-445

The answers are: **441-C; 442-D; 443-B; 444-D; 445-A. Figure 4.1** is a cross-section through the rostral portion of the **medulla**. Structures found at this level include: A - **restiform body**; B - **nucleus and tractus solitarius**; C - **vestibular nuclei**; D - **medial lemniscus**; E - **pyramids**; F - **inferior olive**; G - **nucleus ambiguus**; and H - **nucleus of cranial nerve XII** (hypoglossal). The portion of the ventricular system seen at this level is the open portion of the **4th ventricle**. The **inferior olive** (F) is probably the most distinctive structure seen in cross-section at this level of the brainstem. The pathway responsible for carrying proprioceptive information from the spinal cord is the **medial lemniscus** (D). The origin of most of the axons found in the **pyramids** (E) is from the motor and premotor cortices of the frontal lobes as well as from primary sensory cortex (postcentral gyrus). The **nucleus ambiguus** (G) provides axons that are carried by cranial nerve X (as well as cranial nerves IX and XI) for innervation of the muscles of the soft palate, pharynx and larynx.

Items 446-450

Examination of a 35-year-old man reveals that he has a severe impairment of visual acuity, blurring of vision and diplopia. The patient has pronounced weakness of all four extremities, the deep tendon reflexes are exaggerated and he has bilateral Babinski's signs. The patient complains of feelings of numbness and tingling in the extremities, trunk and face. He also describes a sensation of 'electricity' on passive or active flexion of the neck. Examination reveals impairment of vibratory, position and pain sensation in the extremities. The nurse states that the man has urinary incontinence. The patient's speech is slurred and somewhat slow and has a sing-song quality (scanning speech). On attempting to stand and walk, the patient shows tremors and incoordination of the muscles of the trunk and extremities and ataxia of gait. The patient states that his symptoms were not always as severe as they are now, but they tended to vary in nature and severity over a number of years.

446. Given these signs and symptoms, the **MOST** likely diagnosis might be

   (A)   multiple sclerosis
   (B)   Huntington's chorea
   (C)   tabes dorsalis
   (D)   Friedreich's ataxia
   (E)   Parkinson's disease

447. The patient's slurred speech and scanning speech are **MOST** indicative of damage to the

   (A)   anterior limb of the internal capsule
   (B)   pyramids and pyramidal decussation
   (C)   posterior columns and posterior column nuclei
   (D)   caudate nucleus and putamen
   (E)   cerebellum or its connections with the deep cerebellar nuclei

448. The patient's impairment of vibratory and position sense are **MOST** indicative of damage to the

(A) corticospinal tract
(B) spinothalamic tract
(C) pyramids
(D) spinocerebellar tracts
(E) posterior columns

449. The patient's exaggerated deep tendon reflexes and bilateral Babinski's signs are **MOST** indicative of damage to the

(A) spinocerebellar tracts
(B) posterior columns
(C) corticospinal tracts
(D) spinothalamic tracts
(E) lower motor neurons

450. The blurred vision and diplopia might indicate damage to the

(A) corticospinal tracts
(B) medial longitudinal fasciculus
(C) medial lemniscus
(D) superior colliculus
(E) tractus solitarius

ANSWERS AND TUTORIAL ON ITEMS 446-450

The answers are: **446-A; 447-E; 448-E; 449-C; 450-B. Multiple sclerosis** is primarily a disease of the white matter and is classified as an autoimmune disease resulting in demyelination. The signs and symptoms of multiple sclerosis are so diverse that their enumeration would include all of the symptoms which can result from injury to any part of the neuraxis from the spinal roots to the cerebral cortex. Moreover, the signs and symptoms vary in nature and severity with the passage of time. **Retrobulbar neuritis** is a very common manifestation of multiple sclerosis leading to a profound loss of visual acuity. Diplopia in multiple sclerosis may be caused by involvement of the **medial longitudinal fasciculus** resulting in an internuclear ophthalmoplegia. Involvement of the pyramidal tracts gives rise to spasticity, hyperreflexia and bilateral Babinski's signs. Weakness of the extremities is the most common sign of the disease and may be manifested as monoplegia, hemiplegia, paraplegia or quadriplegia. The cerebellum or its connections with the brainstem are involved in the majority of cases giving rise to **speech disturbances** (slurred and scanning speech), **ataxia** of gait, tremors and incoordination of the muscles of the trunk and extremities. Urinary disturbances are also common, including

incontinence. Damage to the posterior columns produces **paresthesias** including spontaneous feelings of numbness and tingling in the extremities, trunk or face.

Items 451-454

The neuroradiologist asks you to compare normal with abnormal arteriograms of the circle of Willis and cerebral arterial supply. You correctly note that the abnormal film shows a complete occlusion of the right internal carotid artery where it lies within the cavernous sinus.

Choose the **BEST** response.

451.   One of the symptoms shown by the patient with the abnormal film is blindness in the right eye. This is due to compromise of which branch of the internal carotid artery?

    (A)   lenticulostriate
    (B)   ophthalmic
    (C)   middle cerebral
    (D)   anterior cerebral
    (E)   posterior communicating

452.   The branch of the internal carotid artery which provides **MOST** of the blood supply to the lateral aspect of the frontal and parietal lobes is the

    (A)   anterior cerebral
    (B)   middle cerebral
    (C)   posterior cerebral
    (D)   superior cerebellar
    (E)   basilar

453.   Occlusion of which artery would **MOST** severely compromise the blood supply to the visual cortex?

    (A)   posterior cerebral
    (B)   middle cerebral
    (C)   anterior cerebral
    (D)   ophthalmic
    (E)   internal carotid

454.   The oculomotor nerve passes between which two arteries at the base of the brain and may be affected by an aneurysm of either of these arteries?

   (A)   middle cerebral - anterior cerebral
   (B)   anterior cerebral - anterior communicating
   (C)   superior cerebellar - anterior inferior cerebellar
   (D)   posterior cerebral - superior cerebellar
   (E)   basilar - vertebral

ANSWERS AND TUTORIAL ON ITEMS 451-454

The answers are: **451-B; 452-B; 453-A; 454-D**. One of the first major branches of the internal carotid artery is the **ophthalmic artery** which in turn gives rise to the **central retinal artery**. Occlusion of either the ophthalmic or its branch, the central retinal artery, could result in **blindness**. The vessels which provide most of the blood supply to the lateral aspects of the frontal and parietal lobes of the cerebral hemispheres are the **middle cerebral arteries**. The posterior cerebral arteries provide most of the blood supply to the occipital lobes which are the location of the visual cortices. The **oculomotor nerve** (CN III) exits the brainstem between the posterior cerebral and the superior cerebellar arteries and thus an aneurysm of either artery could compromise the nerve.

A 57-year-old man was admitted to the emergency room complaining of sharp pains in his lower extremities. He described the pains as being like 'jabs of lightning' or the 'stick of a sharp needle'. He stated that the pains would come and go over the past three years but they have become more frequent during the last few months. On testing it is noted that the man walks with an uncertain gait, shows an incoordination in the movements of the legs and a noticeable slapping of the feet. The patient shows Romberg's sign. Deep tendon reflexes at the ankle and knee are absent and the patient lacks vibratory and position sense in both lower extremities. Muscle strength appears to be normal. Cranial nerves appear intact but the pupils of both eyes are constricted, fail to respond to light but show normal reaction to accommodation-convergence. When queried about previous illness, the patient admits to having had syphilis when he was younger.

Choose the **BEST** response.

455. Given these symptoms and description, the **MOST** likely diagnosis would be

   (A)   syringomyelia
   (B)   multiple sclerosis
   (C)   amyotrophic lateral sclerosis
   (D)   tabes dorsalis
   (E)   Friedreich's ataxia

456. The pupillary responses shown by this patient might indicate a lesion in the

   (A)   lateral geniculate nucleus
   (B)   nucleus of Edinger-Westphal
   (C)   pretectal region
   (D)   cranial nerve III
   (E)   Meyer's loop

457. The loss of vibratory and position sense in this patient are explainable by damage to the

   (A)   ventral roots
   (B)   posterior roots and posterior columns of the spinal cord
   (C)   lateral white column of the spinal cord
   (D)   anterior white commissure of the spinal cord
   (E)   corticospinal tracts

458. A patient with Romberg's sign would show

    (A)   a tendency to sway and fall when asked to stand with the feet together and the eyes closed
    (B)   a dorsiflexion of the large toe and a fanning of the lateral four toes
    (C)   inability to touch the tip of the nose with the index finger
    (D)   inability to correctly determine a figure such as a numeral drawn on the skin by the examiner
    (E)   loss of pain and temperature sensation from the affected part of the body

459. The **MOST** likely explanation for the ataxia in this patient is

    (A)   loss of ventral horn motor neurons
    (B)   damage to the cerebellum
    (C)   loss of position sense in the affected extremities
    (D)   loss of descending input from the cerebral cortex
    (E)   loss of lateral horn motor neurons

ANSWERS AND TUTORIAL ON ITEMS 455-459

The answers are: **455-D; 456-C; 457-B; 458-A; 459-C**. The triad of symptoms - lancinating or lightning pains, ataxia, and dysuria together with the triad of signs - **Argyll-Robertson pupils**, absence of deep tendon reflexes and the loss of proprioception are characteristic of **tabes dorsalis** (progressive locomotor ataxia). Tabes is a late manifestation of **neurosyphilis** and is characterized pathologically by degenerative changes in the posterior roots, in the posterior funiculi of the spinal cord and in the brainstem. The destruction of the posterior roots explains the lancinating pains felt by these patients. Later, destruction of the posterior columns accounts for the loss of reflexes and the appearance of **Romberg's sign** (with eyes closed and feet together, the patient will sway and fall). Destruction of the posterior columns also accounts for the loss of vibratory and position sense and leads to ataxia in the patient. Involvement of the pretectal region of the midbrain accounts for the Argyll-Robertson pupil.

A 40-year-old woman complains that for several months she has had a weakness in both of her hands. When she accidentally burned her hand on a hot iron she felt no pain. Neurological examination reveals signs of wasting of the small muscles of both hands and loss of pain and temperature sensation in the cervical and upper thoracic dermatomes in a shawl-like distribution, with prominent loss of pain and temperature sensation in the hands and forearms. Deep tendon reflexes are absent in the arms.

Choose the **BEST** response.

460.   Which of the following diagrams of spinal cord cross-sections **MOST** accurately depicts the location and extent of the damage in this woman?

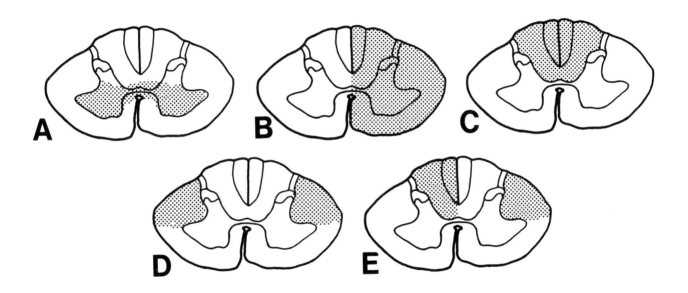

Figure 4.2

461.   One likely diagnosis for this patient given the signs and symptoms is

   (A)   poliomyelitis
   (B)   Horner's syndrome
   (C)   cerebrovascular accident
   (D)   cervical syringomyelia
   (E)   carotid aneurysm

462. Wasting of the small muscles of the hand is **MOST** likely due to damage or destruction of the

   (A)   corticospinal tracts
   (B)   rubrospinal tracts
   (C)   spinothalamic tracts
   (D)   ventral horn motor neurons
   (E)   posterior columns

463. The bilateral loss of pain and temperature sense is **MOST** likely due to damage or destruction of the

   (A)   anterior white commissure
   (B)   spinothalamic tract
   (C)   corticospinal tract
   (D)   posterior columns
   (E)   ventral horn motor neurons

ANSWERS AND TUTORIAL ON ITEMS 460-463

The answers are: **460-A; 461-D; 462-D; 463-A**. The patient shows the classical and most common form of **syringomyelia**. This is a disease of the spinal cord of unknown cause and is characterized pathologically by gliosis and cavitation of variable extent. This disease most often affects the **cervical region** of the cord (cross-section A in **Figure 4.2**) but may affect the lumbar cord and lower medulla as well. Patients experience loss of pain and temperature sensation due to destruction of the pain fibers crossing through the anterior white commissure. As the cavitation increases, the ventral horn motor neurons will be affected leading to atrophy of the denervated muscles. Atrophy of the small muscles of the hand localize the lesion in this patient to spinal segments C8 and T1. The loss of reflexes is probably due to the destruction of the posterior root collaterals to the ventral horn motor neurons and to loss of the motor neurons themselves.

A 51-year-old women presents with a partial weakness of the muscles of the right side of her face, conjunctivitis and a corneal ulcer on the same side. On testing, it is found that she has cutaneous hypesthesia of the right side of her face and loss of the corneal reflex on the right side. Further testing shows that she also has a complete loss of response to caloric stimulation on the right and a horizontal nystagmus. Auditory testing reveals she has nerve deafness in the right ear. Following lumbar puncture, her CSF shows an increased protein content and skull X-rays reveal an enlargement of the internal acoustic meatus. A CT scan shows displacement and rotation of the fourth ventricle and changes in the cerebellopontine angle.

Choose the **BEST** response.

464.   Given these signs and symptoms, the **MOST** likely diagnosis would be

   (A)   multiple sclerosis
   (B)   Friedreich's ataxia
   (C)   Korsakoff's syndrome
   (D)   tic douloureux
   (E)   acoustic neuroma

465.   The loss of the caloric response and nystagmus indicate involvement of the

   (A)   superior colliculus
   (B)   medial geniculate body
   (C)   vestibular portion of cranial nerve VIII
   (D)   trigeminal nerve
   (E)   facial nerve

466.   The absence of the corneal reflex and hypesthesias of the face indicate involvement of the

   (A)   trigeminal nerve
   (B)   facial nerve
   (C)   vagus nerve
   (D)   glossopharyngeal nerve
   (E)   chorda tympani

467. Another deficit that this patient may show with careful testing is loss of taste on the anterior 2/3 of the right side of the tongue. This is explainable by damage to cranial nerve

    (A)   VIII
    (B)   VII
    (C)   IX
    (D)   X
    (E)   XII

ANSWERS AND TUTORIAL ON ITEMS 464-467

The answers are: **464-E; 465-C; 466-A; 467-B**. **Tumors of cranial nerve VIII** account for about 10 percent of all intracranial tumors and probably arise in the Schwann cell sheath of the nerve. These tumors grow slowly and symptoms are usually present for many months or years before the diagnosis is made. Damage to the auditory portion of cranial nerve VIII results in loss of hearing from the affected ear. The tumor frequently arises along the nerve in the internal acoustic meatus which accounts for the enlargement of the meatus seen in an X-ray. As the tumor enlarges, it compresses surrounding structures and affects nearby cranial nerves. Compression of the brainstem results in the distortion of the 4th ventricle and cerebellopontine angle as seen in the CT scan. The loss of the response to **caloric stimulation** and the **horizontal nystagmus** are due to destruction of the vestibular portion of nerve VIII. The trigeminal nerve is affected in 50% of the cases and results in the loss of sensation and loss of the corneal reflex on the same side as the tumor. Cranial nerve VII (facial) passes through the internal acoustic meatus along with cranial nerve VIII, and thus is frequently involved. Damage to cranial nerve VII results in paralysis or weakness of the facial muscles, loss of tearing from the ipsilateral eye and diminished taste sensation from the ipsilateral side of the tongue (anterior 2/3). The conjunctivitis and corneal ulcers are due to drying of the eye and the inability to close the eyelids (paralysis of the orbicularis oculi muscle).

Items 468-471

A newborn infant, on gross examination, has an obvious spina bifida in the lumbar region with meningomyelocele and hydrocephalus. X-ray (ventriculography) and CT examination reveal enlargement of the lateral ventricles, and shows that the 4th ventricle lies at the level of the foramen magnum.

Choose the **BEST** response.

468. Spina bifida is defined as

   (A) a failure of formation of the meninges
   (B) a failure in the closure of the spinal column due to a defect in the development of vertebrae
   (C) a failure of the proper formation of spinal nerve roots
   (D) an enlargement of the ventricular system of the brain
   (E) a failure of neural tube morphogenesis

469. The position of the 4th ventricle at the level of the foramen magnum indicates

   (A) The infant has a perfectly normal ventricular system.
   (B) The infant has herniation of the brainstem and cerebellum through the foramen magnum (Arnold-Chiari malformation).
   (C) There is blockage of the ventricular system at the interventricular foramina.
   (D) There is a defect in the occipital bone of the skull.
   (E) There is a defect in the articulation between the atlas and the skull.

470. The term meningomyelocele indicates that

   (A) The spinal cord and nerve roots are intact and only a herniated meningeal sac is present.
   (B) The lumbar vertebrae lack a neural arch but the spinal cord and spinal nerve roots are intact and no meningeal sac is present.
   (C) A portion of the spinal cord has been distorted, the spinal nerve roots are stretched and the cord is in a superficial position in the herniated meningeal sac.
   (D) The central canal of the spinal cord has become enlarged.
   (E) The ventricular system of the brain has become enlarged.

471. This child would likely exhibit all of the following **EXCEPT**:

   (A)   normal cutaneous and proprioceptive sensation in the lower extremities
   (B)   loss of deep tendon reflexes in the lower extremities
   (C)   urinary incontinence
   (D)   weakness or paralysis of the leg muscles
   (E)   atrophy of leg muscles

ANSWERS AND TUTORIAL ON ITEMS 468-471

The answers are: **468-B; 469-B; 470-C; 471-A. Spina bifida** is a failure in the closure of the spinal column due to a defect in the development of vertebrae. It may be classified as spina bifida occulta, spina bifida with meningocele or spina bifida with meningomyelocele depending on the severity of the involvement of the meninges, spinal cord and nerve roots. **Spina bifida occulta** indicates a simple defect only in the closure of the vertebrae. **Meningocele** indicates the presence of a sac-like protrusion of skin and meninges while **meningomyelocele** indicates the presence of a sac containing spinal cord and nerve roots. With the meningomyelocele defect in the lumbar region as this child shows, the signs and symptoms include: weakness and atrophy of leg muscles, disturbances of gait, urinary incontinence, loss of deep tendon reflexes of the legs and impairment of cutaneous and proprioceptive sensations in the lower extremities. The **Arnold-Chiari malformation** is a herniation of the brainstem and cerebellum through the foramen magnum and has a relatively high occurrence rate with cases of spina bifida with meningomyelocele.

A 48-year-old man of Norwegian extraction complains of 'pins and needles' tingling sensations in all four extremities. He also states that on occasion he feels shooting pains in the arms and legs and a pressure sensation in the abdomen. The man walks with an unsteady, uncoordinated gait. On testing it is found that there is loss of vibratory and position sense in both lower extremities. Both pain and temperature sensation appear to be normal. There is noticeable muscular weakness in both lower limbs. Deep tendon reflexes are absent in the lower limbs but appear normal for the upper limbs. Bilateral Babinski's sign can be elicited and the patient has a positive Romberg's test. Other laboratory tests reveal that the patient has primary anemia (vitamin B_{12} deficiency).

Choose the **BEST** response.

472.   Which of the following diagrams of spinal cord cross sections would **MOST** likely represent the extent of damage in this patient?

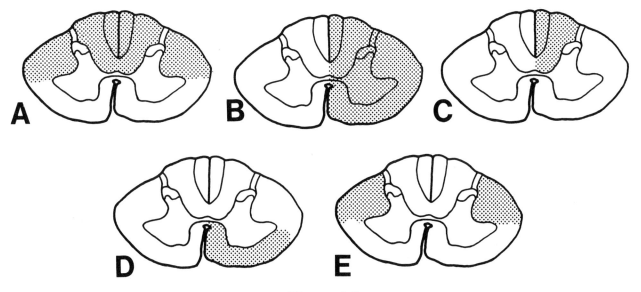

Figure 4.3

473.   A patient with Babinski's sign would exhibit

(A)   A tendency to sway and fall when asked to stand with the feet together and the eyes closed.
(B)   A dorsiflexion of the large toe and a fanning of the lateral four toes.
(C)   Inability to touch the tip of the nose with the index finger.
(D)   Inability to correctly determine a figure such as a numeral drawn on the skin by the examiner.
(E)   Loss of pain and temperature sensation from the affected part of the body.

474. The loss of vibratory and position sense is indicative of damage to the

   (A)   spinothalamic tracts
   (B)   spinocerebellar tracts
   (C)   posterior columns
   (D)   corticospinal tracts
   (E)   rubrospinal tracts

475. The patient's description of shooting pains and the 'pins and needles' sensations are indicative of damage to the

   (A)   spinothalamic tracts
   (B)   corticospinal tracts
   (C)   rubrospinal tracts
   (D)   posterior roots
   (E)   spinocerebellar tracts

ANSWERS AND TUTORIAL ON ITEMS 472-475

The answers are: **472-A; 473-B; 474-C; 475-D**. The neurological manifestations of **pernicious** (primary) **anemia** are degenerative changes in the peripheral nerves and central nervous system. The white matter of the brain appears to be more affected than the gray matter. Peripheral nerves, tracts in the spinal cord and the white matter of the brain all can show varying degrees of degeneration. The constellation of symptoms shown by this patient is termed 'combined system disease' where both the **dorsal columns** and the **lateral corticospinal tracts** are damaged as shown by spinal cord section A in **Figure 4.3**. The characteristic early clinical symptoms are paresthesias in the distal parts of the extremities and a spastic, ataxic weakness of the legs. The presence of the bilateral Babinski's signs in this patient indicates damage to the corticospinal tracts. Normally, when the sole of the foot is stroked firmly, the toes flex (plantar response). However, with damage to the corticospinal tracts, the response of the foot to stroking is extension of the big toe and a fanning of the lateral four toes (**Babinski's sign**). The loss of vibratory and position sense indicates damage to the posterior columns. The 'pins and needles' sensations (paresthesias) indicate damage to the peripheral nerves or nerve roots.

Following occlusion of an artery, a patient has spinal cord damage represented by the shaded portion in **Figure 4.4** below.

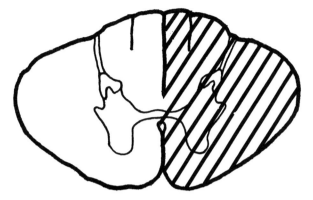

Figure 4.4

Choose the **BEST** response.

476. This spinal cord lesion is known clinically as

   (A) amyotrophic lateral sclerosis
   (B) Friedreich's ataxia
   (C) combined system disease
   (D) tabes dorsalis
   (E) Brown-Séquard syndrome

477. One type of sensory deficit shown by such a patient would include loss of vibratory sensation

   (A) bilaterally in all four extremities
   (B) in the lower extremity contralateral to the lesion
   (C) in the lower extremity ipsilateral to the lesion
   (D) in the upper extremity contralateral to the lesion
   (E) bilaterally in the lower extremities

478. One type of motor deficit shown by such a patient would include

   (A) an ipsilateral upper motor neuron lesion below the level of the cord lesion
   (B) a contralateral upper motor neuron lesion below the level of the cord lesion
   (C) a lower motor neuron lesion in both lower extremities
   (D) an upper motor neuron lesion in both upper extremities
   (E) an upper motor neuron lesion in the contralateral upper extremity

479. One type of sensory deficit in such a patient would include loss of pain and temperature sensation

      (A)   below and contralateral to the cord lesion
      (B)   below and ipsilateral to the cord lesion
      (C)   above and ipsilateral to the cord lesion
      (D)   below and bilaterally
      (E)   in both upper extremities

ANSWERS AND TUTORIAL ON ITEMS 476-479

The answers are: **476-E; 477-C; 478-A; 479-A**. The signs and symptoms associated with hemisection of the cord constitute the **Brown-Séquard syndrome**. Neurological findings include: (1) loss of proprioceptive information carried by the posterior white columns from below the lesion on the same (ipsilateral) side. The posterior columns are the fasciculi gracilis and cuneatus which are comprised primarily of axon collaterals from type I and II dorsal root afferents. These axons carry proprioceptive information such as touch, pressure, vibration, and joint and position sense from the body, particularly from the limbs. (2) an upper motor neuron lesion below the level of the injury on the same side. Spinal hemisection destroys the fibers of the lateral corticospinal tract which originates in large part from the primary motor and sensory cortices of the contralateral cerebral hemisphere. These axons synapse on sensory interneurons and directly on motor neurons. Destruction of these fibers anywhere along their length constitutes an upper motor neuron lesion. (3) loss of pain and temperature sensation below the cord lesion on the opposite (contralateral) side. Spinal hemisection destroys the lateral and anterior spinothalamic tracts which carry pain, temperature and light touch information from the periphery. The axons synapse with interneurons in the substantia gelatinosa and dorsal horn. These axons of the second order neurons cross the midline via the anterior white commissure of the spinal cord, and thus a hemisection produces pain and temperature anesthesia contralateral to the lesion.

A 62-year-old man presents with the classic symptoms of Parkinson's disease. The patient shows a moderate rhythmic tremor in both upper extremities. His face is mask-like (e.g., unexpressive) with few emotional movements. The normal involuntary blinking movements of the his eyes are decreased in frequency. When the patient walks, his head and shoulders are stooped forward and he slowly shuffles his feet. When walking, the patient keeps his arms somewhat extended and adducted and flexed. He does not swing his arms as he walks.

Choose the **BEST** response.

480.   Disease or dysfunction of what structure of the brain has been implicated in Parkinson's disease?

    (A)   pulvinar
    (B)   habenula
    (C)   superior colliculus
    (D)   substantia nigra
    (E)   medial geniculate nucleus

481.   The neural pathway implicated in Parkinson's disease is a dysfunction of the projection of the structure in Item 480 above to the

    (A)   cerebral cortex
    (B)   spinal cord
    (C)   cerebellum
    (D)   superior colliculus
    (E)   corpus striatum

482.   Parkinson's disease is related to dysfunction in the production or release of the neurotransmitter

    (A)   serotonin
    (B)   dopamine
    (C)   acetylcholine
    (D)   norepinephrine
    (E)   adrenalin

483.   The current treatment for Parkinson's disease is to administer the amino acid precursor to the dysfunctional neurotransmitter. The neurotransmitter itself cannot be administered because it

(A)   is toxic to the patient
(B)   cannot be synthesized
(C)   does not cross the blood-brain barrier
(D)   would not have any effect on the disease process
(E)   acts too slowly to be of any benefit

ANSWERS AND TUTORIAL ON ITEMS 480-483

The answers are: **480-D; 481-E; 482-B; 483-C**. **Parkinson's disease** (paralysis agitans) is a complex of symptoms due to widespread, diffuse lesions in the basal ganglia and cerebral cortex and is characterized clinically by a variety of signs, which include a mask-like facial expression, dysarthria, alternating tremor, stooped posture, abnormalities of gait, cogwheel rigidity of the muscles, slowness and poverty of movements, lack of associated movements, disturbances of postural control and symptoms of autonomic nervous system dysfunction. These signs, along with the absence of evidence of pyramidal tract involvement, make a diagnosis conclusive. Parkinson's patients have been shown to have a reduction in the amount of **dopamine** in the corpus striatum and in the substantia nigra. The dopaminergic neurons of the substantia nigra project to the corpus striatum. **L-dopa**, the amino acid precursor to dopamine, is administered to patients because dopamine will not cross the blood-brain barrier.

A 42-year-old woman presents with a sudden hemiplegia and hemianesthesia involving only the right leg. With testing it is found her symptoms also include mental confusion, some clouding of consciousness and aphasia.

Choose the **BEST** response.

484.   Which artery (or major branch) has probably been occluded in this patient?

   (A)   left anterior cerebral
   (B)   right middle cerebral
   (C)   right posterior cerebral
   (D)   right anterior cerebral
   (E)   left posterior cerebral

485.   Concerning cerebral dominance, what can you likely conclude about this patient?

   (A)   She is right hemisphere dominant.
   (B)   Both hemispheres have equal dominance.
   (C)   Neither hemisphere is dominant.
   (D)   Her left hemisphere is dominant.
   (E)   No conclusion can be reached.

486.   If another patient had the **OPPOSITE** artery occluded than the one in the example above, which of the following symptoms probably would **NOT** be seen?

   (A)   hemiplegia only
   (B)   aphasia only
   (C)   hemianesthesia only
   (D)   hemiplegia or hemianesthesia
   (E)   hemiplegia or aphasia

ANSWERS AND TUTORIAL ON ITEMS 484-486

The answers are: **484-A; 485-D; 486-B**. The **anterior cerebral artery** supplies the anterior limb of the internal capsule, the head of the caudate nucleus and the putamen. Its distribution also includes the motor and sensory cortex which controls the legs. Since the corticospinal system decussates in the medulla, occlusion of the left anterior cerebral artery would produce the hemiplegia and hemianesthesia in the right leg. Since the anterior cerebral artery also supplies the white matter deep to **Broca's area**, occlusion of the left artery would also result in the aphasia seen in this patient. Most people (95%) are left cerebral hemisphere dominant, which means the language area, Broca's area, resides in that hemisphere. Thus a patient with occlusion of the right anterior cerebral artery is much less likely to exhibit aphasia.

Items 487-490

A CT scan of a patient reveals damage to the medulla oblongata in the region supplied by the posterior inferior cerebellar artery. The neurologist concludes the patient has a classic Wallenberg's syndrome (lateral medullary syndrome).

Choose the **BEST** response.

487.   The patient would show an ipsilateral Horner's syndrome due to

    (A)   damage to the mammillary bodies
    (B)   destruction of descending sympathetic fibers
    (C)   damage to the inferior olive
    (D)   damage to the superior cervical ganglion
    (E)   damage to the nucleus ambiguus

488.   The patient would show dysphagia and dysarthria due to

    (A)   destruction of the vestibular nuclei
    (B)   destruction of the inferior olive
    (C)   destruction of the nucleus ambiguus
    (D)   damage to the medial lemniscus
    (E)   damage to the pyramids

489.   The patient would show a nystagmus due to

    (A)   damage to the vestibular nuclei
    (B)   damage to the nucleus ambiguus
    (C)   damage to the inferior olive
    (D)   destruction of the superior cerebellar peduncle
    (E)   destruction of the medial lemniscus

490. The patient would have destruction of the spinal trigeminal tract and nucleus. This damage would produce

(A)   cerebellar-type dysfunction in the ipsilateral arm and leg
(B)   impairment of pain and temperature sense in the ipsilateral leg
(C)   impairment of pain and temperature sense on the contralateral side of the face
(D)   impairment of taste sensation on the contralateral side of the face
(E)   impairment of pain and temperature sense on the ipsilateral side of the face

ANSWERS AND TUTORIAL ON ITEMS 487-490

The answers are: **487-B; 488-C; 489-A; 490-E**. The **posterior inferior cerebellar artery**, which arises from the vertebral artery, supplies the lateral area of the medulla oblongata. The signs and symptoms that result from occlusion of this artery are called the lateral medullary syndrome or **Wallenberg's syndrome**. These signs and symptoms would include: dysphagia and dysarthria due to weakness of the ipsilateral palatal and laryngeal muscles (innervated by fibers originating in the nucleus ambiguus); impairment of pain and temperature sensation on the contralateral side of the body due to destruction of the ascending spinothalamic tracts; impairment of pain and temperature sense on the ipsilateral side of the face due to destruction of the spinal trigeminal nucleus and tract; nystagmus due to damage to the vestibular nuclei; cerebellar dysfunction in the ipsilateral arm and leg due to damage to the inferior cerebellar peduncle and the cerebellum. The patient would show ipsilateral **Horner's syndrome** due to destruction of the descending sympathetic fibers. The symptoms of Horner's syndrome would include decreased sweating on the face, flushed face due to vasodilation, and ptosis of the upper eyelid.

A 53-year-old female patient has evidence of both a lower motor neuron lesion and an upper motor neuron lesion due to an expanding tumor in the spinal cord.

Choose the **BEST** response.

491.   Characteristics of an upper motor neuron lesion include all of the following **EXCEPT**:

      (A)   Babinski's sign
      (B)   exaggerated deep tendon reflexes
      (C)   hypertonia
      (D)   spastic paralysis
      (E)   astereognosis

492.   Characteristics of a lower motor neuron lesion include all of the following **EXCEPT**:

      (A)   Babinski's sign
      (B)   flaccid paralysis
      (C)   hypotonia
      (D)   hyporeflexia
      (E)   muscle atrophy

493.   Upper motor neuron lesions involving the spinal cord can be produced by damage to the

      (A)   spinothalamic tract
      (B)   posterior columns
      (C)   corticospinal tract
      (D)   spinocerebellar tracts
      (E)   Lissauer's tract

494.   Lower motor neuron lesions are produced by damage to the

      (A)   corticospinal tract
      (B)   rubrospinal tract
      (C)   ventral horn motor neurons
      (D)   dorsal root ganglia
      (E)   spinocerebellar tracts

495. In addition to injury to the spinal cord as in the example above, damage to which of the following structures would also result in a lower motor neuron lesion?

(A)   caudate nucleus
(B)   substantia nigra
(C)   red nucleus
(D)   vestibular nuclei
(E)   nucleus of the facial nerve

ANSWERS AND TUTORIAL ON ITEMS 491-495

The answers are: **491-E; 492-A; 493-C; 494-C; 495-E**. A **lower motor neuron lesion** is defined as damage to the 'final common pathway', i.e., the motor neurons that synapse directly with skeletal muscle. In the spinal cord, lower motor neurons are the ventral horn motor neurons, but lower motor neurons also include neurons of cranial nerve nuclei (such the facial nerve nucleus) that innervate muscles of the head and neck. Damage to lower motor neurons causes a flaccid paralysis or paresis, decreased muscle tone (hypotonia), decreased reflexes (hyporeflexia) and eventual wasting or atrophy of the muscle.

Upper motor neurons are defined as those neurons and axons of the corticospinal, corticopontine and corticobulbar tracts. A lesion to the upper motor neurons that influence the spinal cord will cause a spastic paralysis or paresis, hyper-reflexia of the deep tendon reflexes, reduced or absent abdominal reflexes, hypertonia, **Babinski's sign** and the clasp-knife reaction.

Items 496-500

Match the brain region listed below with the most appropriate description of that region or structures found within the region in the numbered items that follow. Answers may be used once, more than once, or not at all.

(A)   Diencephalon
(B)   Midbrain
(C)   Pons
(D)   Upper medulla
(E)   Lower medulla

496.   Location of the major structure involved in reflexive orientation of the eyes and the head to visual stimuli.

497.   Location of the decussation of the corticospinal tract.

498.   Location of the second order neurons that receive direct synapses from axons of the posterior column of the spinal cord.

499.   Location of the motor nucleus for the muscles of facial expression.

500.   Location of the portion of the ventricular system called the cerebral aqueduct.

ANSWERS AND TUTORIAL ON ITEMS 496-500

The answers are: **496-B; 497-E; 498-E; 499-C; 500-B.** The **superior colliculus**, which receives direct visual input from the optic tracts, is responsible for orientation of the eyes and head to visual stimuli. The superior colliculi are located in the **tectum** of the midbrain and are the larger of the four swellings called the **corpora quadrigemina**. The portion of the ventricular system found in the midbrain is the **cerebral aqueduct**. The tectum forms the roof for the cerebral aqueduct while the tegmentum of the midbrain forms the floor. The nucleus of the facial nerve (cranial nerve VII) which provides axons that innervate the muscles of facial expression, is found at the level of the pons. Both the dorsal (posterior) column nuclei and the pyramidal decussation are found at the level of the caudal end of the medulla. The dorsal column nuclei include the **nucleus gracilis** which receives axons from the fasciculus gracilis of the spinal cord and the **nucleus cuneatus** which receives axons from the fasciculus cuneatus of the spinal cord. The dorsal column nuclei constitute the second order neurons which convey **proprioceptive information** from the extremities to the thalamus. The **corticospinal tracts** originate from the primary motor and sensory cortices of the cerebrum and pass through the entire brainstem on their way to the spinal cord. Approximately 85-90% of the axons of the each corticospinal tract decussate within the caudal medulla to continue as the **lateral corticospinal tract** of the cord. The other 10-15% remain ipsilateral as the **anterior corticospinal tract**.

248

A 57-year-old man presents with paralysis and atrophy of the ipsilateral half of the tongue, paralysis of the contralateral arm and leg and impairment of tactile and position sensation in the trunk and extremities on the paralyzed side.

Choose the **BEST** response.

501.   The site of the lesion that would produce these symptoms would **MOST** likely be the

    (A)   spinal cord
    (B)   lateral portions of midbrain
    (C)   medial region of the medulla oblongata
    (D)   lateral portions of the pons
    (E)   midline of the cerebellum

502.   The paralysis of the contralateral arm and leg is **MOST** likely due to damage to the

    (A)   spinothalamic tracts
    (B)   medial lemniscus
    (C)   inferior olive
    (D)   middle cerebellar peduncle
    (E)   pyramidal tracts

503.   The impairment of tactile and position sense contralateral to the lesion is **MOST** likely due to damage to the

    (A)   pyramidal tracts
    (B)   inferior olive
    (C)   middle cerebellar peduncle
    (D)   medial lemniscus
    (E)   nucleus ambiguus

504.   The paralysis and atrophy of the tongue is **MOST** likely due to damage to the

    (A)   nucleus ambiguus
    (B)   spinal trigeminal nucleus
    (C)   facial nucleus
    (D)   hypoglossal nucleus
    (E)   medial lemniscus

ANSWERS AND TUTORIAL ON ITEMS 501-504

The answers are: **501-C; 502-E; 503-D; 504-D**. This patient exhibits a vascular lesion involving the medial portions of the **medulla (medial medullary syndrome)**. The paramedian area of the medulla is nourished by perforating branches which arise from the **vertebral arteries**. Occlusion of one of these vessels would produce a lesion involving the pyramids and since the pyramids contain the descending **corticospinal tracts**, such a lesion would give rise to an upper motor neuron deficit of the contralateral extremities.

Involvement of the **medial lemniscus** would result in loss of proprioceptive information (tactile and position sense) from the contralateral portion of the body. The medial lemnisci are comprised of axons originating in the dorsal column nuclei (nucleus cuneatus and gracilis). Involvement of the hypoglossal nucleus and/or the hypoglossal nerve fibers exiting the brain stem would give rise to the paralysis and atrophy of the ipsilateral half of the tongue. The **hypoglossal nucleus** lies in the dorsal aspect of the medulla just deep to the fourth ventricle. The axons descend through the medulla to exit the brainstem between the inferior olivary nucleus and the pyramids.

Items 505-508

A 33-year-old woman complains of double vision and a drooping of her upper eyelids. She states that, initially, the visual problems and drooping were transient, but they are now constant. When she speaks, it is noted that her voice is nasal and weak, and with prolonged talking, her voice fatigues to the point of unintelligibility. She states that her throat becomes tired when she eats a large meal. Her face shows little movement and when she attempts to smile, her expression resembles a snarl more than a smile. As she speaks, she holds a hand under her jaw. Blood tests reveal the patient has a abnormally high serum titer of antibodies to human acetylcholine receptors.

Choose the **BEST** response.

505.   The diagnosis for this patient is **MOST** likely to be

    (A)   Raynaud's disease
    (B)   Parkinson's disease
    (C)   Weber's syndrome
    (D)   myasthenia gravis
    (E)   Reye's syndrome

506. The symptoms shown by this patient are the consequence of a

(A)   loss of acetylcholine receptors at the neuromuscular junction
(B)   lesion within the caudate nucleus
(C)   lesion within the red nucleus and substantia nigra
(D)   loss of skeletal muscle fibers
(E)   loss of ventral horn motor neurons

507. Innervation of the skeletal muscle that raises the upper eyelid is by cranial nerve

(A)   III
(B)   VII
(C)   V
(D)   IV
(E)   VI

508. The clinician orders a CT scan of the mediastinum for this patient because

(A)   there may be an aneurysm of the aortic arch
(B)   the patient may have left ventricular hypertrophy
(C)   the thymus gland may have some pathogenetic role in this patient's disease process
(D)   there may be an esophageal stenosis or atresia
(E)   there may be a congenital heart defect

ANSWERS AND TUTORIAL ON ITEMS 505-508

The answers are: **505-D; 506-A; 507-A; 508-C**. This patient suffers from **myasthenia gravis** which is characterized by weakness and undue fatigability with exercise or muscular use. It most frequently affects the oculomotor, facial, laryngeal, pharyngeal, proximal limb and respiratory muscles. The facial muscle involvement gives rise to a characteristic smile call the 'myasthenic snarl'.

Myasthenia gravis is an **autoimmune syndrome** that results in the loss of **acetylcholine receptors** from the postsynaptic membrane of the neuromuscular junction. It has been demonstrated that 85% of patients have circulating antibodies against human acetylcholine receptors. The thymus gland appears to play an as yet unidentified pathogenetic role in myasthenia gravis. While a CT scan of the mediastinum is not a diagnostic test, 65% of patients with this disease have thymic hyperplasia and 10% have thymomas.

A 17-year-old boy was working as a caddie when he was struck by a golf ball on the right side of the temple just above and in front of the ear. The boy was transported unconscious to the hospital. In the hospital emergency room, the boy regained consciousness for a brief period, but then lapsed into unconsciousness again. On examination, the right pupil was dilated and there was decreased muscle tone in the left leg. A Babinski's reflex was elicited from the left leg but not from the right. Lumbar puncture revealed an increased CSF pressure and some blood in the CSF. A skull radiograph revealed a compressed fracture of the anterior, inferior angle of the parietal bone.

Choose the **BEST** response.

509.   The **MOST** likely diagnosis of this patient is

   (A)   subdural hematoma
   (B)   contusion of the cervical spinal cord
   (C)   extradural hemorrhage
   (D)   Arnold-Chiari malformation
   (E)   occlusion of the cerebral aqueduct

510.   If your diagnosis includes rupture or tearing of a blood vessel, which vessel or one of its branches is **MOST** likely damaged in this patient?

   (A)   middle meningeal artery
   (B)   middle cerebral artery
   (C)   superior sagittal sinus
   (D)   vertebral artery
   (E)   internal carotid artery

511.   What portion of the brain is injured to account for the hemiplegia and Babinski's sign on the left side?

   (A)   left medulla oblongata
   (B)   right occipital lobe
   (C)   right precentral gyrus
   (D)   left temporal lobe
   (E)   right pons and cerebellum

512. Damage to which cranial nerve would explain the dilated pupil?

(A) right trochlear nerve
(B) left trigeminal nerve
(C) left optic nerve
(D) right oculomotor nerve
(E) right optic nerve

513. What test would you employ to detect possible blockage of the subarachnoid space?

(A) Weber's test
(B) Romberg's test
(C) Allen's test
(D) Tinel's test
(E) Queckenstedt's test

ANSWERS AND TUTORIAL ON ITEMS 509-513

The answers are: **509-C; 510-A; 511-C; 512-D; 513-E**. This patient has a right-sided **extradural hemorrhage** due to fracture of the **parietal bone** in the region of the pterion. The anterior division of the **middle meningeal artery** (and vein) passes directly beneath this portion of the skull and is in danger of tearing with a fracture. The initial trauma is responsible for the patient being found unconscious, but recovery of consciousness for a period only to relapse into unconsciousness is characteristic of such injuries. The relapse is due to the accumulation of a large **blood clot** (hematoma) between the skull and the dura mater. The hematoma places pressure on the right precentral gyrus of the cerebrum and causes the hemiplegia and Babinski's sign on the left side. The expanding blood clot probably places indirect pressure on the right oculomotor nerve which is responsible for the dilated pupil on the right side. The clot is also responsible for the raised cerebrospinal fluid pressure. **Queckenstedt's test** (compressing the internal jugular vein and observing CSF pressure changes) is used to detect blockage of the subarachnoid space. Blood in the CSF is probably due to a small leakage from the extradural space into the subarachnoid space at the fracture site.

Figure 4.5 below represents the visual pathways. The labeled bars represent regions where damage has occurred to the visual pathways. Use Figure 4.5 to answer the items that follow. Answers may be used once, more than once, or not at all.

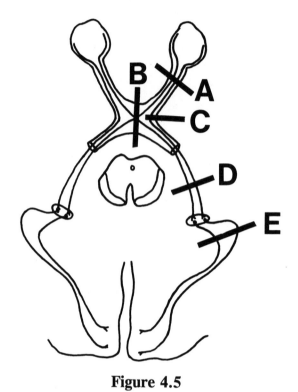

Figure 4.5

514. Which of the lesions above would produce a left temporal and right nasal hemianopia?

(A)　A
(B)　B
(C)　C
(D)　D
(E)　E

515. Which of the lesions above would produce a bilateral homonymous hemianopia?

(A)　A
(B)　B
(C)　C
(D)　D
(E)　E

516. Which of the lesions above includes the portion of the optic radiations called Meyer's loop?

(A)   A
(B)   B
(C)   C
(D)   D
(E)   E

517. Which of the following representations of the visual fields corresponds to a lesion at E.

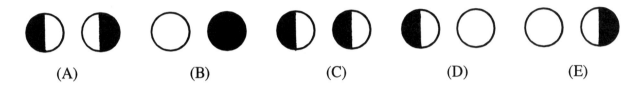

(A)   (B)   (C)   (D)   (E)

518. Which of the following representations of the visual fields corresponds to a lesion at A.

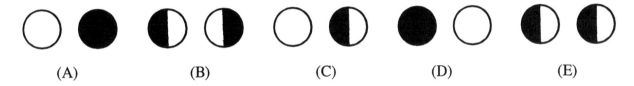

(A)   (B)   (C)   (D)   (E)

ANSWERS AND TUTORIAL ON ITEMS 514-518

The answers are: **514-D; 515-B; 516-D; 517-C; 518-A**. **Figure 4.5** shows the **visual pathways**. Axons within the optic nerves partially decussate at the **optic chiasm** with axons originating from the temporal retina remaining ipsilateral while those originating from the nasal retina cross at the chiasm to synapse in the contralateral **lateral geniculate nucleus** (LGN). From the LGN, axons travel as the optic radiations to synapse mainly within the **primary visual cortex (Area 17 of Brodmann)**. A complete lesion of the optic nerve (point A) would produce a total blindness in the affected eye. A lesion that involves one optic tract (point D) would produce a **heteronymous hemianopia** (left temporal and right nasal hemianopia with a lesion of the right optic tract). A lesion that involved only the decussating fibers of the optic chiasm (point B) would produce a **bilateral homonymous hemianopia**. A portion of the optic radiations called **Meyer's loop** (point D) extends into the temporal lobe and carries axons representing the superior visual quadrants.

Figure 4.6 is a coronal section through the brain.

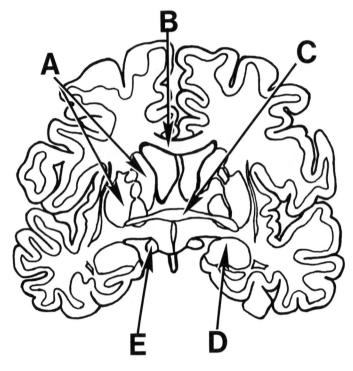

Figure 4.6

519.   Structure which represents the amygdala.

    (A)   A
    (B)   B
    (C)   C
    (D)   D
    (E)   E

520.   Fiber bundle that interconnects the rostral portions of the temporal lobes.

    (A)   A
    (B)   B
    (C)   C
    (D)   D
    (E)   E

521. Fiber bundle that contains efferents of retinal ganglion neurons.

    (A)   A
    (B)   B
    (C)   C
    (D)   D
    (E)   E

522. The structure labeled at B represents a large fiber bundle called the

    (A)   internal capsule
    (B)   anterior commissure
    (C)   fornix
    (D)   corpus callosum
    (E)   pyramidal decussation

523. The structures labeled at A are sometimes referred to collectively as the

    (A)   corpus striatum
    (B)   insula
    (C)   island of Reil
    (D)   corpora quadrigemina
    (E)   trigone

ANSWERS AND TUTORIAL ON ITEMS 519-523

The answers are: **519-D; 520-C; 521-E; 522-D; 523-A**. **Figure 4.6** is a coronal section of the brain through the level of the **anterior commissure**. Structures labeled are: A - **head of caudate nucleus** and **putamen** (corpus striatum); B - **corpus callosum**; C - **anterior commissure**; D - **amygdala**; E - **optic tract**. The head of the caudate nucleus and the putamen/globus pallidus complex are frequently referred to as the **corpus striatum**. The anterior commissure is composed of commissural fibers interconnecting the rostral portions of the temporal lobes. The optic tracts contain efferent axons from the retinal ganglion cells. The anterior limb of the internal capsule lies at the level of the anterior commissure and divides the head of the caudate nucleus from the lenticular nucleus. The amygdala is a large nucleus that lies in the rostral pole of the temporal lobe and is considered part of the **limbic system**.

A 39-year-old woman was seen by the neurologist after fainting and remaining unconscious for several hours. When consciousness returned, she appeared confused and was unable to speak. Examination revealed a spastic paralysis of her right arm but no atrophy. Her right leg and both left extremities appeared normal. Her tongue protruded to the right but was not atrophic. Her right facial muscles were paralyzed, but only those below the eye. There were no apparent deficits in pain or temperature or other somesthetic modalities. There appeared to be no visual defects. The medical history of this patient revealed she had suffered from subacute bacterial endocarditis about a year and a half prior to the present situation.

Choose the **BEST** response.

524. Given these signs and symptoms, the **MOST** likely diagnosis for this patient is embolism

    (A)   at the origin of the right internal carotid artery
    (B)   in the basilar artery
    (C)   in the superior sagittal sinus
    (D)   in a branch of the left middle cerebral artery
    (E)   in the right middle cerebral artery

525. Which of the following diagrams would **MOST** accurately depict the extent of the lesion in this patient?

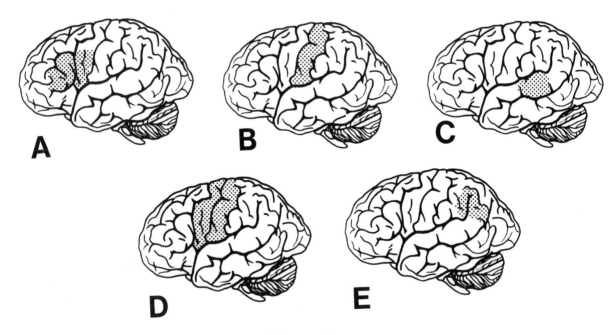

Figure 4.7

526. Which of the following is the **MOST** likely explanation for the lower facial paralysis in this patient?

    (A)   The portion of the facial nucleus controlling the lower face receives a bilateral cortical projection while the portion controlling the upper face receives only a contralateral cortical projection.

    (B)   The entire facial nucleus receives only a contralateral cortical projection.

    (C)   The entire facial nucleus receives a bilateral cortical projection.

    (D)   The entire facial nucleus receives only an ipsilateral cortical projection.

    (E)   The portion of the facial nucleus controlling the upper face receives a bilateral cortical projection while the portion controlling the lower face receives only a contralateral cortical projection.

527. The speech deficit seen in this patient is called

    (A)   alexia without agraphia

    (B)   Wernicke's aphasia

    (C)   Broca's aphasia

    (D)   alexia with agraphia

    (E)   conduction aphasia

ANSWERS AND TUTORIAL ON ITEMS 524-527

The answers are: **524-D; 525-D; 526-E; 527-C**. The **spastic paralysis** of only the right upper extremity suggests damage to a restricted portion of the **cerebral cortex**. A lesion of the subcortical white matter, internal capsule or cerebral peduncle would most likely have resulted in paralysis of the lower extremity as well. A lesion within the internal capsule would also have produced sensory deficits not seen in this patient. Upper motor neuron deficits of both the tongue and the face further support this contention. The portion of the facial nucleus that controls the upper facial muscles receives a bilateral projection from the motor cortex while the portion of the nucleus controlling the lower facial muscles receives a contralateral projection only. Thus, with cortical damage, facial paralysis is evident only in those muscles below the eye. The presence of Broca's (motor) aphasia further localizes the damage to the frontal opercular area of the dominant (usually left) hemisphere. An **embolism** in a branch of the **left middle cerebral artery** would produce the signs and symptoms seen in this patient. Emboli in the arterial supply to the brain are common sequelae in patients with a history of **bacterial endocarditis**.

Items 528-533

Figure 4.8 is a lateral view of the brain. Match the labeled structures with the description in the items below. Answers may be used once, more than once, or not at all.

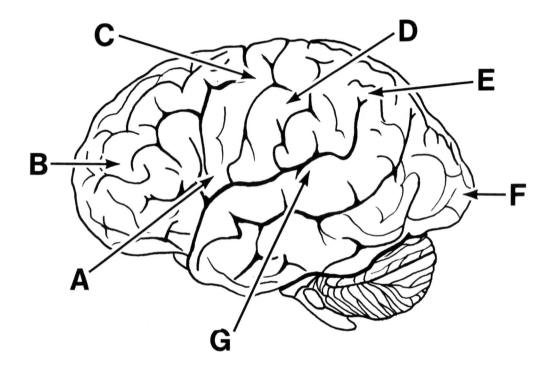

Figure 4.8

528. Region of cerebral hemisphere where damage would produce the loss of ability to read (alexia) and write (agraphia).

529. Region of cerebral hemisphere that receives direct connections from the lateral geniculate nucleus of the thalamus.

530. Region of the cerebral hemisphere where damage would result in Wernicke's aphasia.

531. Region of the cerebral hemisphere that would control volitional movement of the hand and fingers.

532. Region of the cerebral hemisphere known as the primary somesthetic area or Brodmann's areas 3, 1 and 2.

533. Region of the cerebral hemisphere known as the primary auditory cortex.

ANSWERS AND TUTORIAL ON ITEMS 528-533

The answers are: **528-E; 529-F; 530-G; 531-A; 532-D; 533-G**. **Figure 4.8** shows a lateral view of the left hemisphere of the brain. Labeled areas are: A - **upper extremity portion** of the precentral gyrus (**primary motor cortex**, Brodmann's area 4); B - **frontal cortex**; C - **precentral gyrus** (primary motor cortex, Brodmann's areas 4); D - **primary sensory cortex** (Brodmann's areas 3, 2 and 1); E - **angular gyrus** (Brodmann's area 39); F - **primary visual area** (Brodmann's area 17); G - **primary auditory area** (Brodmann's area 41 and 42, Wernicke's area). The angular gyrus is the caudal part of the inferior parietal lobule and is interconnected with the supramarginal gyrus and Wernicke's area. It also receives connections from the areas 17, 18 and 19. A lesion of this area in the dominant hemisphere results in the loss of ability to read (alexia) and write (agraphia). The primary visual cortex (area 17) receives direct connections from the lateral geniculate nucleus of the thalamus. A lesion of the primary auditory cortex (areas 41 and 42, Wernicke's area) in the dominant hemisphere causes a fluent, paragrammatical aphasia (also known as auditory receptive or sensory aphasia). The precentral gyrus which contains the primary motor cortex is responsible for initiation of voluntary movement of skeletal muscles of the limbs. The postcentral gyrus (primary somesthetic area) receives pain, temperature and other somesthetic information relayed from certain thalamic nuclei.

Items 534-537

At autopsy, the pathologist explains that the patient, a 5-year-old child, had a medulloblastoma that appeared to have arisen in the vermis of the cerebellum and had invaded the 4th ventricle and the neighboring cerebellar hemispheres.

Choose the **BEST** response.

534.   When alive, this child would have shown all of the following signs and symptoms **EXCEPT**:

   (A)   astereognosis
   (B)   ataxia
   (C)   intention tremor
   (D)   nystagmus
   (E)   wide-based stance

535. Other signs or symptoms of cerebellar disease include all of the following **EXCEPT**:

(A) dysdiadochokinesia
(B) decomposition of movement
(C) scanning speech
(D) hypotonia
(E) paralysis

536. The cerebellum probably receives input from all of the following structures or areas **EXCEPT**:

(A) vestibular nuclei
(B) hippocampus
(C) pontine nuclei
(D) motor and premotor cortex
(E) spinal cord

537. Efferents from the cerebellum project directly to all of the following **EXCEPT**:

(A) dentate nuclei
(B) lateral geniculate nuclei
(C) globose nuclei
(D) emboliform nuclei
(E) fastigial nuclei

ANSWERS AND TUTORIAL ON ITEMS 534-537

The answers are: **534-A; 535-E; 536-B; 537-B**. Disorders of the **cerebellum** result in distinctive symptoms and signs and can often be localized to specific portions of the cerebellum. The most common lesion involving the vestibulocerebellum (vermis and flocculonodular lobe) is the **medulloblastoma**, a rapidly growing tumor usually occurring in childhood and usually fatal within a year. Involvement of the fourth ventricle would result in increased intracranial pressure and internal hydrocephalus. Patients with cerebellar disease would not show loss of stereognosis since this information is carried to the thalamus via the medial lemniscal system. Patients with cerebellar disease have considerable loss of muscular coordination but would not show paralysis. The hippocampus is part of the limbic system and probably has no connections with the cerebellum. The Purkinje cells of the cerebellum project directly to the four **deep cerebellar nuclei** - the dentate, globose, emboliform and fastigial nuclei.

A 45-year-old woman states that she has suffered from headaches for several months. She now complains of double vision. Lately she has noticed that her left arm seems weak and she has become increasingly more clumsy with her left hand (e.g., dropping dishes and other small items). On examination, her left ankle and knee deep tendon reflexes were exaggerated and a Babinski's sign was elicited on the left. An eye examination revealed that her right pupil was larger than the left and her right eye was turned outward and downward. When asked to look at an object placed close to her nose, her right eye did not converge and neither a light nor an accommodation reflex could be elicited from the right eye. The muscles of the right side of her face below the eye were paralyzed and when asked to protrude her tongue, it deviated to the right.

Choose the **BEST** response.

538.   A CT scan showed this patient to have a tumor. Given these signs and symptoms, where would you expect this tumor to lie?

   (A)   caudal medulla at the level of the pyramidal decussation
   (B)   rostral medulla at the level of the obex
   (C)   at the level of the cerebral peduncle near the emergence of the right oculomotor nerve.
   (D)   cerebellopontine angle
   (E)   sella turcica

539.   The origin of the axons which control pupillary constriction with light stimulation and during accommodation are found in the

   (A)   lateral geniculate nucleus
   (B)   superior colliculus
   (C)   nucleus of the trochlear nerve
   (D)   nucleus solitarius
   (E)   nucleus of Edinger-Westphal

540.   The facial paralysis and tongue paralysis in this patient are **MOST** likely due to damage to the

   (A)   hypoglossal nerve directly
   (B)   facial nerve directly
   (C)   corticobulbar fibers to the nuclei of the facial and hypoglossal nerves
   (D)   medial lemniscus
   (E)   medial longitudinal fasciculus

541. Preganglionic parasympathetic nerve fibers carried by the oculomotor nerve synapse in the

(A) ciliary ganglion
(B) otic ganglion
(C) superior cervical ganglion
(D) pterygopalatine ganglion
(E) nodose ganglion

ANSWERS AND TUTORIAL ON ITEMS 538-541

The answers are: **538-C; 539-E; 540-C; 541-A**. This patient exhibits the signs and symptoms of hemiplegia alternata oculomotoria, or **Weber's syndrome**. This can be caused by a vascular lesion to the midbrain or by a tumor adjacent to the cerebral peduncle and the emergence of the oculomotor nerve (cranial nerve III). The facial paralysis and tongue paralysis are both due to damage to the descending corticobulbar fibers that innervate the nuclei of the facial and hypoglossal nerves. Damage to the oculomotor nerve produces ptosis of the eyelid and paralysis of all the extrinsic muscles of the eye except the superior oblique and the lateral rectus (which explains the position of the eye in this patient). The oculomotor nerve also carries the preganglionic parasympathetic nerve fibers which originate in the **nucleus of Edinger-Westphal** and synapse in the ciliary ganglion. The postganglionic fibers innervate the ciliaris muscles and the sphincter pupillae. Damage to these fibers results in pupillary dilation and the lack of response of the pupil to light or accommodation.

Items 542-544

A 41-year-old homeless man was admitted to the emergency room exhibiting confusion, disorientation, amnesia and confabulation. During a lucid period, the man admitted that he drank a large amount of cheap wine and he had done so for years. Alcohol was found in the patient's blood and also in the CSF following a spinal tap. The patient showed a paralysis of both lateral recti, horizontal and vertical nystagmus and a paralysis of conjugate gaze. He also had weakness of the legs, foot drop and ataxia in walking. The muscular weakness appeared to be greatest in the distal parts of the lower limbs. Reflexes were absent at the ankle and knee, the plantar response was absent and the abdominal skin reflexes were decreased. There was anesthesia in the distal part of his lower limb and vibratory and kinesthetic sensibilities were impaired. The nerves of his lower limbs were sensitive to pressure and the muscles were painful when squeezed.

Choose the **BEST** response.

542. The peripheral nerve disturbances in this patient are classified as

   (A)   polyneuritis
   (B)   tabes dorsalis
   (C)   combined system disease
   (D)   myasthenia gravis
   (E)   pseudobulbar palsy

543. The mental symptoms shown by this patient are classified as

   (A)   Froehlich's syndrome
   (B)   amyotrophic lateral sclerosis
   (C)   Paget's disease
   (D)   Hurler's syndrome
   (E)   Korsakoff's syndrome

544. The mental symptoms shown by this patient suggest lesions within the limbic system of the brain. The limbic system would include all of the following **EXCEPT**:

   (A)   hippocampus
   (B)   cerebellum
   (C)   cingulate gyrus
   (D)   mammillary bodies
   (E)   amygdaloid nuclei

ANSWERS AND TUTORIAL ON ITEMS 542-544

The answers are: **542-A; 543-E; 544-B**. Alcohol-vitamin deficiency polyneuritis is the most common form of neuritis and occurs in patients addicted to the use of large amounts of **alcohol** and who have associated nutritional deficiencies. The pathology of polyneuritis is due mainly to a noninflammatory degeneration of the peripheral nerves producing the pains, paresthesias, weakness and sensory loss. Muscular weakness is usually greatest in the distal part of the extremities. The confusion, disorientation, amnesia and confabulation seen in this patient are referred to as **Korsakoff's syndrome**. Patients with Korsakoff's syndrome exhibit pathological changes in diencephalic structures that are part of the limbic system. Typically, they have damage to the mammillary bodies as well as the medial dorsal nucleus of the thalamus. The cerebellum is not classified as part of the limbic system.

Items 545-549

Figure 4.9 is a transverse MRI image of the normal brain.

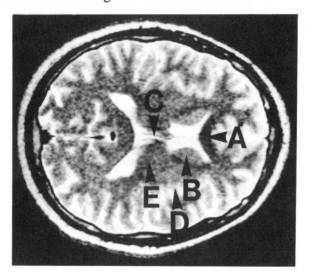

Figure 4.9

545.   Region of the brain were a lesion would result in damage to the hippocampus.

546.   Region of the brain which is divided into the rostrum, genu, body and splenium.

547.   Portion of the ventricular system that extends into the infundibulum and tuber cinereum.

548.   Region of the brain where the internal structures include the nucleus ventralis posterolateralis.

549.   Region of the brain which is a part of the basal ganglia.

Figure **4.10** is a MRI scan of a midsagittal slice through the head.

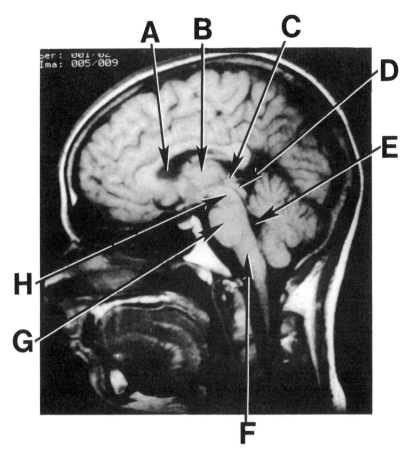

Figure 4.10

550. The corpora quadrigemina which function to control visual and auditory reflexes.

551. CSF exits here into the subarachnoid space via the foramen of Magendie and foramina of Luschka.

552. Site of tumor of the pineal gland which could compress aqueduct of Sylvius.

553. Region of the brain that is described as the major sensory relay nucleus of the brain.

554. Vascular accident here could compromise the red nucleus and substantia nigra.

555. Location of the principal sensory nucleus which gives origin to the fibers of the trigeminal nerve.

ANSWERS AND TUTORIAL ON ITEMS 545-549

The answers are: **545-D; 546-A; 547-C; 548-E; 549-B. Figure 4.9** is a transverse MRI image through the third ventricle and thalamus. Labeled structures are; A - **corpus callosum**; B - **head of caudate nucleus**; C - **third ventricle**; D - **temporal lobe**; E - **thalamus**. A lesion of the temporal lobe would result in damage to the hippocampus. The corpus callosum is comprised of axons interconnecting the cerebral hemispheres and is divided into the rostrum, genu, body and splenium. The genu of the callosum is shown in A. The 3rd ventricle, which lies between the two halves of the thalamus, has an extension that descends into the infundibulum of the pituitary. The nucleus ventralis posterolateralis is one of a number of nuclei which make up the thalamus. The head of the caudate nucleus is seen in this scan and it plus the putamen and globus pallidus, comprise the major portion of the basal ganglia.

ANSWERS AND TUTORIAL ON ITEMS 550-555

The answers are: **550-D; 551-E; 552-C; 553-B; 554-H; 555-G. Figure 4.10** is a magnetic resonance image (T1 MRI) of a midsagittal section through the head. Labeled structures are: A - **lateral ventricle**; B - **thalamus**; C - **pineal gland**; D - **tectum of midbrain**; E - **4th ventricle**; F - **medulla**; G - **pons**; H - **tegmentum of midbrain**. The roof of the cerebral aqueduct is known as the tectum and consists primarily of the corpora quadrigemina, the superior and inferior colliculi. **Cerebrospinal fluid** (CSF) circulates throughout the ventricular system of the brain. Three foramina in the roof of the 4th ventricle (foramen of Magendie and foramina of Luschka) allow the CSF to enter the subarachnoid space. A tumor of the pineal gland (C) may compress the anterior portion of the tectum and occlude the aqueduct of Sylvius causing an internal hydrocephalus. The thalamus (B) is the major sensory relay nucleus of the brain, receiving all sensory information except olfactory. The red nucleus and the substantia nigra are part of the extrapyramidal motor system and are large nuclei found within the tegmental region of the midbrain. The principle sensory nucleus of cranial nerve V (trigeminal nerve) lies within the pons and the fibers of the trigeminal nerve exit the brain stem from the lateral portion of the pons.

A 5½-year-old boy was brought to the emergency room by his parents. They said their son had complained earlier of a headache and a stiff neck. During the night he had a fever, had vomited and had a seizure. On examination, the neck stiffness persisted, the neck was tender to the touch and it was very difficult for the examiner to flex the neck muscles. On attempting to flex the head, there was a flexion of the legs at the knees. When the thigh was flexed, it was extremely difficult to extend the leg completely due to pain in the back. The boy seemed to be lethargic, delirious and almost in a stupor. The boy's temperature was 102° F. The boy showed no evidence of cranial nerve palsies or focal neurological signs.

Choose the **BEST** response.

556.   Given these signs and symptoms, the **MOST** likely diagnosis is

  (A)   epidural hematoma
  (B)   meningitis
  (C)   cerebrovascular accident
  (D)   intracerebral tumor
  (E)   epilepsy

557.   In this patient, when the neck was passively flexed, flexion of the leg occurred. This is known as

  (A)   Allen's test
  (B)   Brudzinski's sign
  (C)   Tinel's sign
  (D)   Kernig's sign
  (E)   Trendelenburg's sign

558.   The analysis of the CSF and CSF pressure of this patient would **MOST** likely show all of the following **EXCEPT**:

  (A)   increased white blood cell content
  (B)   increased protein levels
  (C)   clear and colorless consistency to the CSF
  (D)   increased CSF pressure
  (E)   presence of microorganisms

559. Normally in these patients, CSF is obtained

(A) from the lateral ventricles
(B) from the cisterna magna
(C) from the central canal
(D) from the superior sagittal sinus
(E) by lumbar puncture

560. When this patient was on his back and his thigh was flexed on the trunk, extension of the leg was nearly impossible due to back pain. This is known as

(A) Kernig's sign
(B) Trendelenburg's sign
(C) Tinel's sign
(D) Brudzinski's sign
(E) Allen's test

ANSWERS AND TUTORIAL ON ITEMS 556-560

The answers are: **556-B; 557-B; 558-C; 559-E; 560-A**. There are several causes of **meningitis** but the signs and symptoms are basically the same. The onset of meningitis is accompanied by chills and fever, headache, nausea and vomiting, pain in the back and stiffness of the neck. Mental confusion and stupor may occur and convulsive seizures are common. The temperature is usually elevated to 101° to 103° F. There is rigidity of the neck and the patient usually shows both a positive **Kernig's** and **Brudzinski's sign**. A lumbar puncture is done and the laboratory data show increased CSF pressure, and the fluid is cloudy or purulent and contains many leukocytes. The protein content is increased, the sugar content is decreased and organisms can be seen in stained smears of the fluid and can be cultured on the appropriate media.

INDEX

A

B-C

D

L-N

O-R

S

T